Drug Metabolism and Alcohol

Drug Metabolism and Alcohol

A Survey of Alcohol-Drug Reactions —
Mechanisms, Clinical Aspects, Experimental Studies

R.C. Pirola

M.D. (NSW), F.R.A.C.P. Specialist Gastroenterologist,
The Prince Henry, Prince of Wales and Eastern Suburbs Hospitals,
and Department of Medicine, The University of New South Wales, Sydney.

With 16 figures and 15 tables

UNIVERSITY PARK PRESS
Baltimore   •   London   •   Tokyo

DRUG METABOLISM AND ALCOHOL

ISBN 0-8391-1228-9

First Printing

University Park Press

International Publishers in Science and Medicine

233 East Redwood Street
Baltimore, Maryland 21202

to Mavis — who helps me to dream impossible dreams

Foreword

To find a treatise which covers research, theoretical background and practical application for the treatment of patients, is to discover an unusual book indeed. Such a text is particularly needed in the field of alcoholism and drug abuse where only recently have collections been made of papers and articles which usually deal with only one particular and limited aspect of the problem. Dr Romano Pirola is to be congratulated on his outstanding skill in bringing together such a wealth of recent contributions to our knowledge and understanding of the complex effects of alcohol and its interaction with a variety of drugs.

Dr Pirola has been known for years as a distinguished internist and gastroenterologist, interested in the complications of alcoholism, particularly those involving the pancreas. After fine clinical training in Australia, Dr Pirola gathered five years of postgraduate experience in London with Professor Sheila Sherlock and in New York, at the Mount Sinai School of Medicine of the City University of New York and the Bronx Veterans Administration Hospital. Over the last decade Dr Pirola has brought to bear his investigative mind and his broad experience on the general effects of alcohol in the body, including total body metabolism and in particular interaction between ethanol and drug metabolism. This is socially a most relevant concern since, except perhaps in a few aboriginal tribes of Dr Pirola's homeland, alcohol is by far the most widely abused drug in contemporary societies.

Whereas most studies have focused thus far on specific effects of alcohol (i.e. on the intestine, pancreas, liver, brain etc.), Dr Pirola discusses some heretofore neglected aspects of alcoholism — its impact on total body metabolism.

A major characteristic of our modern society is the widespread use and abuse of a variety of pharmacological agents taken for their tranquillising, stimulating or placebo effects. The action of these drugs can be profoundly affected by the acute or chronic intake of alcohol. The stimulation by chronic alcohol consumption of the activity of the hepatic microsomal enzymes which detoxify a variety of drugs may result in decreased effectiveness of important medications such as anticoagulants or sedatives. Conversely, alcohol by its presence may compete with some drugs for a partially common detoxification process in the liver, thereby resulting in enhanced drug retention and increased blood levels with potentially dangerous effects. The increasing number of suicides achieved by the combination of barbiturates and alcohol illustrate the potential danger of the combination of ethanol and other drugs. Another example is the rather striking increase in lethal road accidents in North America and other countries of Western civilisation; this seems to be due not only to enhanced alcohol consumption but also the increased drug use and the potentiation of the alcohol and drug effects, be it through additive and synergistic actions on the central nervous system or through mutual reduction in rates of metabolism and thereby rates of disappearance. The patient given some tranquillisers, if not warned by his physician of this potentially dangerous combination, may after some otherwise acceptable drinking, find himself faced with rather unsuspected potent drug and alcohol effects which deprive him of his normal ways of coping with driving or other responsibilities.

Dr Pirola's dissertation is a timely account for the physician of the manner in which alcohol and drugs interact. It also gives us rational concepts and ingenious hypotheses to explain many of these clinically important drug interactions. A book such as this has been long overdue in our modern alcohol- and drug-ridden society. Because of his extensive clinical expertise and his broad training in clinical medicine and pharmacology, Dr Pirola was unusually well prepared to undertake the task of writing this book. It is, therefore, no surprise that he has presented us with a fine and concise treatise which will be read with profit by the clinician as well as the investigator. It is worth pointing out that this book should not only be greatly appreciated by active workers in the field of alcoholism, but that it deserves a much wider audience because the subject touches every physician and health professional.

The reader will find Dr Pirola's pragmatic and critical approach very stimulating and his book extremely well documented. To write the foreword for such a book is a unique privilege indeed; it is with great personal satisfaction that I congratulate my esteemed friend and colleague on this fine achievement.

Charles S. Lieber

Acknowledgements

In writing this book, I have drawn very heavily on the ideas of Professor Charles S. Lieber and on his outstanding contributions to the study of ethanol metabolism. I am also grateful for the helpful discussions with colleagues of Professor Lieber, notably Miss Leonore De Carli, and Drs. Enrique Baraona and Jean-Gil Joly, and in particular for the detailed comments of Dr. Rolf Teschke. The preparation of the manuscript would not have been possible without the help of Mrs Janet Swanson. Acknowledgements to authors and publishers for permission to reproduce or adapt figures and tables from published sources are as follows:

Fig. 1, p.26 (from Mannering; in La Du, Mandel and Way, Fundamentals of Drug Metabolism and Drug Disposition, Williams and Wilkins, Baltimore 1971); Fig. 2, p.32; Fig. 3, p.33 (from Loewy and Siekevitz, Cell Structure and Function, 2nd ed, Holt Rinehart and Winston Inc., New York 1969); Fig. 4, p.35 (from Evans et al.: Brit. Med. J. 2: 485, 1960); Fig. 6, p.68 (from Teschke et al.: Biochem. Biophys. Res. Comm. 49: 1187, 1972); Fig. 7, p.83 (from Lieber: New Eng. J. Med. 288: 356, 1973b); Fig. 9, p.93 (from Misra et al.: Am. J. Med. 51: 346, 1971); Fig. 10, p.94 (from Lieber; in Mule and Brill, Chemical and Biological Aspects of Drug Dependence, Chemical Rubber Company Press, Cleveland, Ohio 1972b); Figs. 11 and 12, p.97; Fig. 13, p.98 (from Pirola and Lieber: Pharmacology 7: 185, 1972); Table II, p.19; Table III, p.20 (from Williams: Gut 13: 579, 1972); Table IV, p.27 (modified from Mannering; in

La Du, Mandel and Way, Fundamentals of Drug Metabolism and Drug Disposition, Williams and Wilkins, Baltimore 1971); Table V, p.40 (from Conney: Pharmacol. Rev. 19: 317, 1967); Table VII, p.58 (from von Wartburg; in Kissin and Begleiter, The Biology of Alcoholism, vol. 1: Biochemistry, Plenum Press, New York and London 1971); Table VIII, p.69 (from Teschke et al.: Arch. Biochem. Biophys. 163: 404, 1974a); Table IX, p.70; Table X, p.71 (from Teschke et al.: Biochem. Biophys. Res. Comm. 60: 851, 1974b); Table XII, p.124; Table XIII, p.127 (from Leake and Silverman; in Kissin and Begleiter, The Biology of Alcholism, vol. 1: Biochemistry, Plenum Press, Oxford and New York 1971); Table XIV, p.128 (from Carroll: Quart. J. Stud. Alc. Supp. 5: 6, 1970).

Contents

1. Introduction

1.1 Ethanol – the Ubiquitous Drug

'It's a good man's failing'
Eugene O'Neill – Long Day's Journey into Night

'Will I have to stop drinking while I'm taking this drug?' That is the question being faced daily by a high percentage, possibly even a majority, of patients for whom drugs are prescribed. The ubiquity of the problem stems from the widespread use (and abuse) of ethanol (ethyl alcohol). From the beginning of recorded time, alcohol intake has been a socially accepted tradition of most societies. Even an 'excessive' intake is commonly viewed with attitudes varying from benign indulgence to grudging admiration. The cocktail party, the wedding reception, the post-examination 'pub-crawl' and the businessman's luncheon are but a few of the many social occasions where there is a definite expectation of the amount and type of alcoholic beverage that will be supplied. Despite the excessive alcohol consumption commonly seen at such a function, the event would lose tremendously if alcoholic drinks were avoided.

In Great Britain in 1970, the average person spent 7% of his total expenditure on alcoholic beverages (McKenzie, 1972). When one allows for the number of people who abstain because of age or other reasons, this figure could become about 14% for the average drinker. Yet the consumption of alcohol in Great Britain is considerably lower than in many other Western countries. In the United States, ethanol is the principal drug of abuse among teenagers (Saltman, 1973). It is estimated that one out of seven male high school students gets drunk at least once a week and over one third get drunk at least four times a year. At the University of California, 43 per cent of male students and 21 per cent of female students had 'one or more problems connected with drinking'. Fifteen per cent of the men and 4 per cent of the women had serious alcohol-related problems. In Australia, Pritchard (1970) estimated that premature death from alcoholism cost the national economy 0.25 per cent of the Gross National Product in lost production alone. To this could be added the appalling costs of alcohol-related road accidents, hospital admissions and crimes. A number of reports indicate that in 8—14 per cent of all Australian hospital admissions, alcohol intake directly contributed to the patient's illness (Wilkinson et al., 1971).

Furthermore, the intake of ethanol in most countries appears to be rising. In Australia, the average consumption of beer rose from 11.7 gallons per year in 1938 to 27 gallons per year in 1970 (Santamaria, 1972). In 1973, the cost of alcoholism in the USA was estimated to have risen by two-thirds, to 25 billion dollars annually, in less than three years (AMA Gazette, 1974). In the same period of time, teenage male drinking rose by over 50 per cent and teenage female drinking by over 100 per cent. Alcoholic pancreatitis, a previously rare disease in Great Britain, is being seen increasingly commonly (Trapnell, 1972). This observation may reflect both the increased total consumption of alcoholic beverages and the fact that the greatest rise has been accounted for by drinks with a higher ethanol content, i.e. wines and spirits rather than beer (McKenzie, 1972).

1.2 The Problem of Assessing Intake

'Are you taking any drugs or medicines?' The clinician who expects a reliable yes or no answer to such a simple question will be sadly misled. Multiple factors are responsible. Few patients seem to intentionally deceive. Some hasten to say no, thinking that the question applies only to drugs of addiction. Some patients on long term therapy with agents such as insulin or hypotensive drugs are so used to their therapy that they seem to no longer class them as 'medicines'. Others may be reticent about mentioning their use of agents such as contraceptive pills or psychotropic or antiepileptic drugs. Still others just forget.

In the case of alcohol, the problem of assessing intake is far greater. There are two main reasons for this. One is that the intake of ethanol tends to be far more variable than that of most other drugs. It will alter from day to day according to innumerable unpredictable social and economic pressures. However, of greater importance is the marked reticence of some people to admit to their true intake. Admittedly, some patients, especially young men, may exaggerate their intake, but the general tendency is to minimise it. This is particularly so in women, some of whom go to great lengths to hide their partiality to alcohol.

1.3 The Growing Problem of Drug Interactions

Drug interactions are an increasingly familiar problem of modern medicine, and of course this includes reactions between alcohol and other drugs. As discussed in an earlier companion volume (Milner, 1972), a particularly dangerous situation exists in the case of the drinking driver who is taking barbiturates, antipsychotics or antianxiety agents. Many drug reactions are unpredictable. Most sensitivity reactions are included in this group. For example, patients given carbamazepine (Tegretol) for trigeminal neuralgia occasionally develop cholestatic jaundice. It is known that carbamazepine can do this, but it is a rare and unpredictable side effect, so a reasonable calculated risk is taken to obtain a therapeutic effect. Such drug reactions are regrettable, but they are just the necessary price we have to pay if we are to use effective drugs at all and not to lapse into therapeutic nihilism. Nevertheless, it is suggested that in the U.S.A., adverse drug reactions annually affect millions of people, cause hospitalization in hundreds of thousands and actual death in tens of thousands (Jick, 1974). What is particularly upsetting is that it is estimated that 70—80% of all drug reactions in hospitals are said to have been predictable (Melmon, 1971). The problem is partly a result of the huge proliferation not only of new drugs, but also of new classes of therapeutic agents. Yesair et al. (1972) estimate that the 195 new single entity drugs introduced in the 10-year period 1961—1970 could theoretically result in 15,000 possible combinations of two drugs. The problem is magnified by the greater efficacy of many new compounds, with the potential for more severe interactions.

This increases the danger of using drugs to treat unrecognised reactions to other drugs, a situation for which Moser (1970) used the phrase 'the domino theory of therapeutics'. Thirty per cent of patients hospitalized for a drug reaction have a further reaction during their admission (Melmon, 1971). In a survey of patients in a general hospital, Hollister (1965) found that those receiving an antibiotic were also given a minimum of 6 and a maximum of 35 other drugs. In another survey of 900 hospitalized patients, Smith et al. (1966) found evidence of drug reactions in 10.8 per cent. Thus there is an increasing tendency for the appearance of articles with such disquieting titles as 'The Diseases Drugs Cause' (Lasagna, 1964) and 'Ill-Health Due to Drugs' (Wilson, 1966). This growing problem is one of the most serious challenges of modern therapeutics. However, there may have been a tendency in recent years to over-react to the situation. Theoretical opportunities for drugs to react with each other are seemingly unlimited. One leading reference book has a tabulated list of possible drug interactions that covers 417 closely printed pages.

Unfortunately, it is impossible to determine the extent to which these theoretical possibilities produce clinically significant harm in practice. Thus it is reassuring to note the conclusions of the Boston Collaborative Drug Surveillance Programme (Jick, 1974). After studying adverse drug effects in 60,000 patients, they concluded that the number of deaths produced was quite small in relation to the number of lives saved by drugs. Unnecessary drug toxicity was present, to some degree, in only one substantial area, namely fluid and electrolyte therapy. There did not appear to be drugs in current use even approximately comparable to thalidomide, with risk grossly out of proportion to benefit. In the Boston study, the frequency of adverse drug reactions for each course of therapy was only 5%. Most of these were minor and of no clinical consequence (nausea, drowsiness, diarrhoea, vomiting and rash). Life-threatening reactions occurred in 0.4% of courses of therapy. These consisted mainly of arrhythmias, bone marrow depression, central nervous system depression, fluid overload and haemorrhage. Drug-attributed deaths occurred in 0.24% of courses of therapy, and half of these were due to hyperkalaemia and/or pulmonary oedema. The magnitude of the problem of drug interactions appears to be largely due to the large number of drugs being prescribed. Other factors, such as dosage, the sever-ity of the illnesses for which the drugs are prescribed, and the presence of renal and hepatic disease are less important. With increasing numbers of drugs given, the frequency of reactions rises disproportionately, indicating that the risks of extra drugs are more than just additive. Polypharmacy has always been a trad-itional feature of medical practice. This was unimportant in the days when drugs were of little value. Unfortunately the greater effectiveness of new compounds has increased, rather than decreased, the pressure on doctors to prescribe more drugs. Thus there is an increasing responsibility for clinicians to familiarise them-selves with the principles of therapeutics and pharmacokinetics and to under-stand the nature and the metabolism of the agents that they prescribe.

Apart from therapeutic agents, life in modern society involves a growing exposure to a variety of other foreign compounds. The list is seemingly endless and constantly expanding. In the home one comes into contact with an increa-sing variety of insecticides, dyes, foodstuff additives, cleaning agents and other compounds, and in some industries the diversity and extent of exposure is even greater. Many of these foreign chemicals enter the body and are handled by drug-metabolizing enzyme systems. Fortunately, health regulations afford some protection from the introduction of potentially toxic compounds but more subtle effects, such as those due to hepatic microsomal enzyme induction are known to occur (see section 4.4.1).

1.4 General Mechanisms of Alcohol-Drug Interactions

There is an almost endless list of possibilities whereby drinking alcoholic beverages can alter the responses to other drugs. Some of the potential mechanisms for these interactions are shown in Table I. Most drug interactions are of two main types:

1) Direct (predominantly acting at the end organ). The administration of one drug alters the relationship between the blood level and the pharmacological response of the other drug.

2) Indirect (predominantly affecting absorption, biotransformation and excretion). The administration of one drug alters the relationship between the blood level and the dosage of the other drug.

An exaggerated pharmacological effect commonly occurs when ethanol is taken at the same time as another drug, as in the case of the enhanced sedation seen in the intoxicated patient taking a barbiturate or phenothiazine. This is partly due to an additive or synergistic effect in the central nervous system. However, in some cases the explanation is a metabolic one due to inhibition of alcohol dehydrogenase or of microsomal pathways of ethanol metabolism. This metabolic inhibition can even be used therapeutically as in the case of ethanol treatment of methanol poisoning, where the major toxic effects of methanol are due to its metabolites. Alcoholism could also cause impaired drug metabolism as a nonspecific result of severe alcoholic liver disease, since any severe generalised disturbance of hepatic function can result in delayed clearance of drugs with more severe and prolonged pharmacological effects (Sherlock, 1968; Zilly et al., 1973). However, the role of hepatic disease in altered rates of drug metabolism is relatively poorly documented. Generally speaking, the handling of drugs by the diseased liver is surprisingly well maintained. Needle hepatic biopsies of patients with hepatitis and cirrhosis show normal activities of microsomal enzymes, except in severe disease (Schoene et al., 1972). The clearance of various drugs in cirrhosis is often normal unless severe hepatic decompensation has developed. Levi et al. (1968) found the half-life of isoniazid to be increased in patients with liver disease, but considered this to be less important than the genetically-determined variation in ability to acetylate this drug. However, severe liver disease could affect drug responses in other ways, for example, by altering rates of absorption, or by altering plasma protein levels and the plasma binding of drugs. If hepatic decompensation supervenes, then the sensitivity of the central nervous system to the same blood levels of drugs may be enhanced, especially in the case of sedatives (Schenker et al., 1974).

The development of tolerance to the action of various drugs, especially sedatives, is another well-known feature of the alcoholic. This may develop at the site of the end-organ when it is loosely referred to as pharmacodynamic tolerance (or central nervous system tolerance when the agent is a sedative). The

Table I. Classification of mechanisms whereby untoward reactions may occur in person drinking alcoholic beverages and taking medications

---

I.   *Direct* (altered response of end organ to same plasma level of medication or of ethanol)

    1.   Pharmacological reaction directly opposed or enhanced.

        a)   by ethanol — see section 7

        b)   by congeners — see section 7.4.1

    2.   Altered responsiveness of end organ directly due to metabolic action of drug — see sections 7.4.3, 8

    3.   Altered responsiveness of end organ due to changes in other organs (e.g. hepatic failure affecting neurological responses) — see section 1.4

II.   *Indirect* (altered plasma level after standard dose)

    1.   Absorption

        a)   Altered gastric emptying — see sections 2.2.5, 2.3.2

        b)   Altered mucosal blood flow — see section 2.2.5

        c)   Altered luminal pH — see section 2.3.3

        d)   Intestinal mucosal damage — see section 2.3.4

        e)   Miscellaneous — see section 2.3.1

    2.   Distribution

        a)   Changes in plasma proteins

            i)   directly due to ethanol — see section 6.6

            ii)   due to alcoholic liver disease — see section 1.4

        b)   Changes in cell uptake

    3.   Metabolism

        a)   Inhibition

            i)   Competitive

                — ADH pathway — see sections 7, 8

                — Microsomal — see sections 6.7, 7

                — Conjugation — see sections 5.9, 7.4.7

            ii)   Non-specific (liver disease) — see section 1.4

        b)   Stimulation

              — ADH pathway — see sections 5.4.1, 6.5.2

             — Microsomal — see sections 4.4, 6.8, 7

    4.   Excretion

---

mechanism or mechanisms underlying pharmacodynamic tolerance are poorly understood. An increased tolerance of the central nervous system to sedatives might conceivably be related to changes in the levels in the brain of tryptophan hydroxylase. This is the rate-limiting enzyme for serotonin synthesis. Its activity is inhibited by the acute administration and enhanced by the chronic intake of either morphine (Knapp and Mandel, 1972) or ethanol (Kuriyama et al., 1971). Pharmacodynamic tolerance can be demonstrated by showing that, for the same blood level of sedative, tolerant animals previously exposed to ethanol show much less sedation and ataxia than controls. This form of tolerance appears to take days to develop. However, an acute form of pharmacodynamic tolerance can appear within hours. Again, the mechanism is not understood. It is best recognised in the case of ethanol; for a given blood level of alcohol, inebriation is greater when the blood ethanol concentration is rising than when it is falling (Harger and Hulpiett, 1956).

Another form of tolerance is drug tolerance. This is also commonly seen in alcoholics and habitual takers of drugs. Comparisons of animals awakening from an anaesthetic dose of a sedative show that animals previously subjected to chronic ethanol intake, and with shortened sleeping times have sedative blood levels similar to those of controls. The mechanism in most cases appears to be an increased rate of drug metabolism in the hepatic smooth endoplasmic reticulum (see section 6.8). However, this same mechanism may have the reverse effect, namely enhanced drug toxicity, if the drug exerts its effects mainly through a metabolite. An example of this is the enhanced susceptibility of alcoholics to carbon tetrachloride toxicity (see section 7.2.6).

Much less is known of the innumerable remaining possible mechanisms for alcohol-drug interactions. Presumably this is partly because theoretical considerations or technical problems make these areas seem to be potentially less fruitful areas for investigation. There are a number of mechanisms whereby the absorption of drugs in alcoholics may be enhanced or impaired. The pharmacological effects of a drug could be increased by the presence of portal-systemic venous shunting (and 'bypass' of the liver) associated with alcoholic liver disease. Even less is known about such possible mechanisms for alcohol-drug interactions as altered transport or storage, impaired mitochondrial function, changes in cell uptake (e.g. due to changes in membrane carriers such as the Y and Z proteins), altered excretion, and the effects of congeners and of associated malnutrition.

It is important to bear in mind that many mechanisms may be involved in the altered pharmacological response to any one drug in the alcoholic. These mechanisms may oppose each other or be additive and the net pharmacological response may vary with such diverse factors as the blood level of alcohol, the duration of drug intake, malnutrition and the presence or absence of hepatic dysfunction. An example of the complexity of the problem is illustrated by the interactions between chlorpromazine and ethanol. As discussed in section 7.3.1, there may be changes in absorption, in distribution, in pharmacodynamic tolerance and in drug tolerance, and the latter may involve at least two possible mechanisms.

2. Absorption

2.1 Normal Drug Absorption

Drugs can be effectively absorbed into the body by a number of routes, including the oral mucosa, the rectum, lungs and skin. However, the traditional and most convenient route of absorption for most drugs is in the gastro-intestinal tract. The various ways in which drugs might cross an epithelial membrane include: simple diffusion through lipoid regions or through aqueous pores of the membrane; filtration through membrane pores; carrier-mediated transport; and vesicular transport, such as pinocytosis. Most drugs are either weak acids or weak bases. Thus the extent to which they are ionised in solution will depend on the pH of the solution and on the pK_a of the drug. Because of their lipid nature, biological membranes are generally permeable to the non-ionised form of a drug but relatively impermeable to the ionised form.

For the most part, absorption of drugs from the gastro-intestinal tract is accounted for by pH dependent, simple non-ionic diffusion across the gastro-intestinal epithelial membrane. This was first demonstrated by a study of the gastric absorption of strychnine and other weak organic bases in the cat (Travell, 1940). Instillation of these compounds into the pylorus-ligated stomach produced no effects when the gastric contents were acid since at low pH the drugs were in a predominantly ionised form. When the stomach contents were made alkaline, the compounds reverted to a predominantly non-ionised form; they were quickly absorbed and the animals died. Over a wide range of pH values, it was shown that the rate of absorption of strychnine was dependent on the concentration of the non-ionised form of the drug. Subsequently, these considerations have been shown to apply to other drugs. At equilibrium, the concentration of the unionised form of any drug will be the same on either side of a lipid mucosal membrane. By altering the pH on one side, the concentration of the unionised form will be increased or decreased (according to whether it is an alkali or an acid) and the absorption will be correspondingly increased or decreased. Thus weak acids such as salicylates and barbiturates are predominantly non-ionised in the stomach and are readily absorbed from the gastric lumen. By contrast, weak bases, such as morphine, ephedrine, quinine and tolazoline are predominantly ionised in the gastric juice. Consequently, their absorption is poor from the stomach and occurs mainly in the intestine.

Gastric absorption of drugs is influenced by other factors apart from the rate of passage across the epithelial membrane. Thus the absorption of salicylates may be enhanced by raising the pH of the gastric juice despite the fact that the drug will then be in a more ionised form. Part of the explanation for this phenomenon may be that (at least in the case of salicylates) alkalinization favours dispersion of the drug and allows a wider mucosal contact to occur. Another explanation may be a faster rate of gastric emptying. Theoretically one might expect that gastric emptying would have opposite effects on the absorption of weak acids and weak bases because of the differences between gastric and intestinal luminal pH. However, the effect of pH is overshadowed by the much larger absorptive surface of the intestine so that, generally speaking, gastric retention markedly reduces drug absorption, regardless of whether the drug is an acid or a base. This probably accounts for much of the impairment of drug absorption associated with eating. In addition, binding of a drug to food or other intestinal contents may also delay absorption. Other factors that are relevant include the solubility of a drug and its concentration.

The intestinal absorption of a drug is affected by pH in the same way as gastric absorption. At the actual site of intestinal absorption, the pH is believed to be about 5.3. Consequently weak bases are better absorbed and weak acids less well absorbed than in the stomach. That intestinal absorption of most drugs involves simple diffusion is indicated by the close correlation between the luminal concentration of the compound and its rate of absorption. A further indication that a simple, non-saturable process is involved is indicated by the failure of drugs to compete with each other for transfer across the epithelium.

That lipid solubility is the physical property determining the speed of transfer of non-ionized molecules across the intestinal epithelium is shown by the parallelism that exists between the rates of absorption of various weak electrolytes and the lipid-to-water partition ratios of their non-ionized form. Thus the absorption of steroids varies with their lipid solubilities. Furthermore, minor structural changes can increase the lipid solubility of a drug and have been shown to correspondingly enhance its absorption.

Completely ionized, lipid insoluble compounds are very poorly absorbed from the gastro-intestinal tract. These include quaternary ammonium compounds such as hexamethonium and aminoglycoside antibiotics such as strepto-mycin. However, therapeutically significant quantities of some of these compounds can be absorbed under certain conditions. In the case of the quaternary ammonium compounds it is postulated that a 'phosphatidopeptide' material derived from the intestinal mucosa may complex with the compounds to facilitate absorption.

2.2 Absorption of Ethanol

2.2.1 Sites

Ethanol is a lipid-soluble non-electrolyte. Hence it can be absorbed from the skin, lungs and all levels of the alimentary tract. Its absorption from the small intestine is extremely rapid. Instillation directly into the duodenum results in blood levels comparable to those obtained by intravenous administration (Davis and Pirola, 1966). These blood levels are much higher than those obtained when the same dose is placed in the stomach of human subjects (Salvisen and Kolberg, 1958), of rats (Haggard and Greenberg, 1940) or of dogs (Payne et al., 1966; Elmslie and Harvey, 1967). However, gastric absorption rates as high as 43% of an administered dose in 20 minutes have been recorded in humans (Hogben et al., 1957).

2.2.2 Luminal Factors

The amount of ethanol absorbed from the stomach is directly related to the gastric luminal concentration (Davenport, 1967). It is not directly related to the luminal pH (Davenport, 1967) nor to the concentration or amount of ethanol in the test meal ingested (Cooke and Birchall, 1969), except in so far as these latter two factors affect the luminal concentration. A number of studies (see Kalant, 1971) have indicated that the overall absorption of ethanol from the alimentary tract is greatest when alcohol is ingested as a 15–30 per cent solution. It is absorbed less rapidly when the ingested concentration is below 10 per cent or over 30 per cent. Delayed absorption after the intake of higher concentrations of ethanol may be due to such factors as dilution due to stimulation of gastric secretion (Chaudhury et al., 1964), delayed gastric emptying (Barboriak and Meade, 1970) and gastric mucosal damage (Chey, 1972). By contrast, a high concentration of ethanol could enhance mucosal blood flow, and this would tend to facilitate the absorption of ethanol (Winne and Remischovsky, 1971).

2.2.3 Type of Alcoholic Beverage

The type of alcoholic beverage also affects the rate of ethanol absorption. From the results of various studies (see Kalant, 1971), the following beverages can be listed in order of decreasing speed of ethanol absorption: wine, gin, whisky and beer. A pure solution of ethanol gives the fastest rate of absorption, so presumably the congeners of alcoholic beverages affect absorption in some way, possibly by altering the rate of gastric emptying.

2.2.4 Effect of Food

That drinking alcohol on an empty stomach speeds its absorption is common knowledge and has been repeatedly confirmed experimentally. The mechanism is mainly the associated delay in gastric emptying, although dilution of ethanol in the stomach presumably plays a role. In addition, the rate of metabolism of ethanol is somewhat faster in the fed than in the fasted state, for reasons that are not clear. The delayed absorption of ethanol with food occurs with all types of foods, particularly with fat. Early reports of increased ethanol absorption after olive oil appear to have been due to the nausea and associated increased gastric emptying produced by this agent.

2.2.5 Effects of Other Drugs

Other drugs can alter the absorption of ethanol in innumerable ways. An accelerated rate of absorption will be produced by any agent that stimulates gastric emptying such as insulin in doses that produce hypoglycaemia (Lolli and Greenberg, 1942) and cholinergic agents (Rinkel and Myerson, 1942). Conversely, alcohol absorption will be retarded by agents that delay gastric emptying such as caffeine (Siegers et al., 1972) or sympathomimetic and anticholinergic drugs (Rinkel and Myerson, 1942). Gastric irritants such as aspirin and pyramidon delay alcohol absorption (Bohmer, 1938; Läuppi, 1954) presumably by causing pylorospasm. However, in ligated intestinal loops (where motility is irrelevant) irritants such as mustard enhance ethanol absorption, apparently as a result of increased mucosal blood flow (Hanzlick and Collins, 1913).

Chlorpromazine could affect ethanol absorption in various ways. Its anti-adrenergic effect might alter gastric emptying and enhance absorption of ethanol. This might account for the accelerated rise in blood alcohol produced by previous chlorpromazine therapy in humans (Sutherland et al., 1960) and in rabbits (Tipton et al., 1961), although, as discussed by these authors, decreased ethanol metabolism may have played a role. In contrast to the above studies, Casier and his colleagues (1966) observed a delay in ethanol absorption after the chronic use of normal therapeutic doses of chlorpromazine, haloperidol and nialamide in human subjects. Differences in dosage may have accounted for the different results obtained by this group. Impaired absorption of ethanol after chlorpromazine was also observed by Jaulmes et al. (1956), but in their study the effect may have been due to a reduction in body temperature associated with simultaneous immersion in water. Elevation of the body temperature, by administration of dinitrophenol, or by external heating, enhances ethanol absorption (Casier and Delaunois, 1943).

Drinking water can also affect ethanol absorption, a point which may be of relevance when one considers that many medications are taken with water. Alcohol absorption is enhanced, at least under certain conditions (Mellanby, 1919), possibly as a result of the stimulation of the emptying of food residue and mucus from the stomach. Ten per cent solutions of $CaCl_2$ (Hanzlick and Collins, 1913) or of $MgSO_4$ (Widmark, 1916) retard the absorption of alcohol. The mechanism is uncertain and Kalant (1971) postulated that retention of water due to $MgSO_4$ and hypomotility due to calcium may play a role.

2.3 Effects of Ethanol on Absorption of Other Drugs

2.3.1 General Considerations

Drinking alcohol could theoretically affect the absorption of other drugs in many ways. However, there is very little known about the clinical relevance of these possibilities. Acute ethanol intake could produce physico-chemical changes in the luminal contents, dilutional effects, altered luminal pH and changes in the motility of the stomach and duodenum. Chronic alcoholism could theoretically alter drug absorption by producing alterations in gastric and intestinal mucosal function (see sections 2.3.3, 2.3.4), changes in bacterial flora, and changes in the secretion of digestive juices. Maddrey and Boyer (1973) found that acute ethanol administration in the rat inhibited bile flow whereas chronic intake enhanced bile flow and bile salt excretion. Ethanol also affects pancreatic secretion (see Pirola and Lieber, 1974) and mesenteric lymphatic flow (Baraona et al., 1973). Drug absorption is probably little influenced by pancreatico-biliary secretion or by mesenteric lymph production. However, a deficiency of the former might conceivably reduce drug absorption secondarily to malabsorption of food, while intestinal lymph flow plays a part in tetracycline absorption (De Marco and Levine, 1969). However, despite these and other (see below) diverse effects of ethanol on alimentary function, there have been few studies into the effects of ethanol on the absorption of other drugs under controlled conditions.

2.3.2 Gastric Emptying

Animal studies have usually (see Barboriak and Meade, 1970) but not invariably (Beazell and Ivy, 1940) indicated that ethanol reduces gastric motility and emptying. Studies in humans have produced more variable results. There have been reports of delayed gastric emptying after ingestion of wine and beer (Barboriak and Meade, 1970), no change after ethanol (Cooke, 1970) and either no change or even an increased emptying after whisky or brandy (Barboriak and Meade, 1970). However, most of these studies employed radiological techniques which are difficult to quantitate. Employing a test meal containing Cr^{51}, and using an external counter of radioactivity, Barboriak and Meade (1970) found a significant delay in gastric emptying after ingestion of 120ml of 100 proof bourbon whiskey. It is possible that some of the reported variations between the results of the above studies are due to differences in the concentrations of ethanol or due to the presence of congeners.

2.3.3 Gastric Acid Secretion

Acute ethanol intake stimulates gastric acid secretion regardless of whether it is given orally or intravenously (Newman and Mehrtens, 1932; Woodward et al., 1957) or applied directly to the fundic mucosa (Davenport, 1967). The stimulation may be partly due to release of gastrin (Cooke and Grossman, 1968; Elwin, 1969a, 1969b).

The effects of chronic ethanol intake on gastric acid secretion are less clear. Some degree of gastritis or of mucosal atrophy is commonly seen in alcoholics, (Chey, 1972). Although the mean maximal acid output of a group of alcoholics in one study was not significantly less than that of controls, those alcoholics who did have biopsy evidence of mucosal atrophy of the body of the stomach did have a marked reduction in maximal acid output (Dinoso et al., 1972). Recently Chey et al. (1972) found that dogs receiving 40 per cent ethanol daily developed a transient increase in maximal acid output. This finding raises the possibility that under some circumstances, chronic ethanol intake could increase the parietal cell mass of the stomach. The relevance of this finding to drinking in humans is uncertain.

2.3.4 Intestinal Damage with Malabsorption in Alcoholics

Malabsorption is common in alcoholics and involves both fat soluble and water soluble components of the diet (see Iber, 1971). Malabsorption of the former could be partly due to hepatic and pancreatic disease. However, malabsorption of water-soluble compounds suggests an intestinal mucosal disturbance. This is commonly attributed to associated malnutrition (Mezey et al., 1970; Halsted et al., 1971). However, recent studies have demonstrated that ethanol itself can produce small intestinal damage in the rat (Baraona et al., 1974). Whatever the mechanism, malabsorption in alcoholics presumably can involve ingested drugs as well as dietary components. Recognition of this possibility could be of importance in the management of the severely ill alcoholic.

2.3.5 Endogenous Intestinal Ethanol

Endogenous ethanol produced in the alimentary tract of mammals appears to result mainly from bacterial activity and fermentation (see section 5.1.7). The amount produced in humans is generally too small to be of significance. However, in one disease, tropical sprue, an increased growth of ethanol-producing coliforms has been demonstrated and it has been postulated that this has a pathogenic role in the production of the associated malabsorption (Klipstein et al., 1973).

3. Drug Metabolism

3.1 Introduction

The terms biotransformation or metabolism are preferable to detoxification since the latter term implies a conversion of a toxic compound to an inactive form. Although this is often the case, the breakdown product may be more pharmacologically active than the parent compound, as in the case of azathioprine (see section 4.3.3), and may be distinctly more toxic as in the case of carbon tetrachloride (see section 7.2.6).

The importance of biotransformation is two-fold. First, it may directly alter the activity of the drug, making it more or less active or completely changing the nature of its action. Second, it may convert a non-polar, lipid-soluble agent into a more water soluble form. Because most drugs are lipid-soluble weak electrolytes, they are readily reabsorbed by the renal tubular epithelium. Thus, renal excretion is favoured by the conversion to a more polar metabolite. Such compounds are less lipid soluble and more ionised and are therefore less able to bind to proteins, to cross cell membranes and to be stored in fat. Thus this type of biotransformation tends to result in inactivation.

Most biotransformations involve enzymatic activity but a small minority occur without enzymatic action. These usually depend only on the presence of certain physico-chemical conditions, such as a change in pH or the presence of macromolecules with which they can react spontaneously. An example of non-enzymatic metabolism is the pH-dependent spontaneous hydrolysis of thalidomide (Williams, 1968). Of course not all drugs undergo biotransformation and thus some are excreted unchanged (at least to some extent). These are usually drugs which are highly polar and therefore not readily metabolized, such as decamethonium and cyclamate. Most drugs can be eliminated by more than one pathway, although for each drug one route of metabolism and excretion may be quantitatively the most important. For example, ethyl alcohol has a major pathway of metabolism, namely alcohol dehydrogenase, but as discussed later, there are other methods of biotransformation of ethanol and in addition some of it is excreted unchanged in breath, faeces and urine. Furthermore the relative quantitative significance of the various pathways can vary considerably in the same person from time to time depending on a large number of physiological, pathological and pharmacological factors. It can also vary between species. Thus amphetamine is predominantly deaminated in the rabbit, but hydroxylated in the dog.

3.2 Phase I and Phase II Reactions

Drug biotransformations generally involve two types of reactions, commonly referred to as phase I and phase II. Phase I or nonsynthetic reactions, involve oxidation, reduction, or hydrolysis. They introduce groups such as OH, COOH, NH_2 and SH into the drug molecule. This can result in increased or decreased activity of the drug or in a qualitative change in its pharmacological properties. Phase II or synthetic reactions involve conjugation. They result in the formation of compounds such as glucuronides and ethereal sulphates and conjugates of amino acids (glycine, glutamine or cysteine) as well as methylation and acetylation reactions. Such conjugations inactivate the drug (or its phase I metabolite) and further reduce its polarity. Examples of these reactions are as follows:

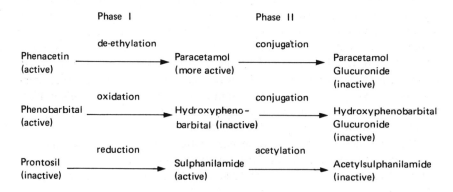

Some drugs are only metabolized by a single phase I reaction (as in the case of trimethadione) or by a series of phase I reactions (as in the case of ethanol). Others are metabolized only by phase II processes:

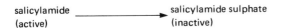

salicylamide   salicylamide sulphate
(active)   (inactive)

3.3 Sites of Drug Metabolism

3.3.1 Relative Importance of Different Organs

The liver is the major site of drug metabolism (table II). Compared to other organs, it is highly active even on a weight for weight basis and when its size and blood flow are taken into consideration, its predominant role can be readily appreciated. However, most tissues have the capacity to biotransform some drugs. This applies especially to the kidneys, intestinal mucosa, lungs and the flora of the gut. Occasionally a tissue has a greater capacity than the liver to metabolize a particular drug, as in the case of the methylation of phenol by the lung. Ethanol is predominantly metabolized in the liver but as discussed in section 5.8 other tissues also have this capacity.

3.3.2 Intracellular Localization

The major site of the biotransformation of many drugs as well as of endogenous substrates such as steroid hormones and lipids appears to be in the

Table II. *In vitro* drug metabolizing activity of various tissues (Williams, 1972)

Tissue	Relative ability to metabolize (hepatic activity taken as 100)			
	Pheno-barbitone	Thio-pentone	Phenol	N-Acetyl-serotonin
Liver	100	100	100	100
Kidney	0	52	48	0
Brain	0	24	3	–
Heart	0	19	0	0
Muscle	0	0	3	–
Small intestine	–	–	3	0
Testis	–	–	6	0
Spleen	–	–	22	0
Lung	–	–	110	0
Adrenal	–	–	13	0

Table III. The location of drug metabolism in the hepatic cell (Williams, 1972)

Fraction of liver homogenate	Relative rate of	
	O-De-ethylation of phenacetin by rabbit liver	O-Demethylation of codeine by rat liver
Whole	100	100
Nuclei (crude)	8	13
Mitochondria	0	0
Microsomes	0	0
Soluble fraction (cytosol)	0	0
Nuclei + soluble	15	26
Mitochondria + soluble	8	0
Microsomes + soluble	85	75

hepatic endoplasmic reticulum. This structure is a diffuse membranous network continuous with the cell membrane, the nuclear envelope and the Golgi apparatus, and may play a role in the transport of materials from one part of the cell to another. After biotransformation in the endoplasmic reticulum, the reaction products are eliminated in bile and urine, but details of the mechanisms responsible are not known. It is possible that the metabolites do not re-enter the cytosol but are transported along the membranes of the endoplasmic reticulum to the cell surface. The ultracentrifugal counterpart of the endoplasmic reticulum is the microsomal fraction. This contains drug metabolizing enzymes but is inactive unless the cell sap or cytosol is added since the latter supplies cofactors such as NADPH (table III). The activity detected in other fractions is usually due to contamination with microsomes due to incomplete separation. When the intact cell is seen under the electron microscope, two types of endoplasmic reticulum can be distinguished. One carries a series of small ribonucleoprotein particles that appear as dots along the membrane giving it a 'rough' appearance, hence the term rough endoplasmic reticulum (RER). This is the major site of protein synthesis. The smooth endoplasmic reticulum (SER) has no attached ribonucleoprotein particles. Drug metabolism takes place predominantly as a result of the activities of the enzymes of the SER, but some drugs are metabolized equally in the RER and the SER. A small minority of drugs are metabolized predominantly by non-microsomal enzyme systems. Notable examples are the cytosolic acetylation of the sulphonamides and of isoniazid.

3.4 Microsomal Drug Metabolism

3.4.1 General Characteristics

Mueller and Miller (1949) provided the first description of the metabolism of a foreign compound by the microsomal fraction of an hepatic homogenate. Subsequently it was found that a number of drugs could be metabolized by a similar hepatic microsomal enzyme system (Brodie et al., 1955). It was found that both the soluble and the microsomal fractions were required, but that the soluble fraction could be replaced by a NADPH generating system consisting of NADP, glucose-6-phosphate (G-6-P) and G-6-P dehydrogenase or simply by NADPH itself. Molecular oxygen was required. The reaction is thus a 'mixed function' oxidase (Mason, 1965) or mono-oxygenase type of reaction (Hayaishi, 1962) since it requires both a reducing agent and molecular oxygen:

$$\text{Drug} - \text{H} + \text{O}_2 + \text{RH}_2 \longrightarrow \text{Drug} - \text{OH} + \text{H}_2\text{O} + \text{R}.$$

Such an enzyme system incorporates only one atom of oxygen from the oxygen molecule into the substrate. The other oxygen atom is reduced to water, the cosubstrate (e.g. NADPH) being used for this purpose. Other functions of this enzyme system include the oxidation of endogenous compounds such as steroids and prostaglandins, the biosynthesis of cholesterol, its catabolism to bile acids and the ω-oxidation of fatty acids.

The microsomal drug metabolizing system displays a versatility that is unique in biochemistry. It is capable of such diverse reactions as deamination, O-, N- and S-dealkylation, hydroxylation of alkyl and aryl hydrocarbons, epoxidation, N-hydroxylation, N-oxygenation, sulphoxidation and the formation of alkylol derivates. This versatility is of considerable biological and pharmacological significance. It provides a rational explanation for some of the widespread changes in drug metabolism that can be produced by single environmental influences or specific disease states. It is also the basis for many of the interactions between drugs (both stimulatory and inhibitory). In the absence of such a versatile system, drug therapy as we know it would be radically different and pharmacological research would be concentrated on the search for drugs utilizing separate and distinct mechanisms of biotransformation. The functions of the microsomal enzymes seem less diverse if one considers them as different types of hydroxylation reactions (Mannering, 1971):

Aromatic hydroxylation
$$CH_3CO - NH - C_6H_5 \xrightarrow{OH} CH_3 - CO - NH - C_6H_4 - OH$$
Aliphatic hydroxylation
$$R - CH_3 \xrightarrow{OH} R - CH_2 - OH$$
N-dealkylation
$$R - NH - CH_3 \xrightarrow{OH} R - NH - CH_2OH \dashrightarrow RNH_2 + CH_2O$$
O-Dealkylation
$$R - O - CH_3 \xrightarrow{OH} R - O - CH_2OH \dashrightarrow ROH + CH_2O$$
Deamination
$$R - CH(NH_2) - CH_3 \xrightarrow{OH} R - C(OH)(NH_2) - CH_3 \longrightarrow R - CO - CH_3 + NH_3$$
Sulphoxidation
$$R - S - R^1 \xrightarrow{OH} R - SOH - R^{1 +} \dashrightarrow R - SO - R^1 + H^+$$
N-oxidation
$$(CH_3)_3N \xrightarrow{OH} (CH_3)_3{}^+ \dashrightarrow (CH_3)_3 NO + H^+$$

As discussed earlier (see section 3.2), there are other mechanisms of drug biotransformation by hepatic microsomes apart from the oxidative and reductive reactions being considered here.

The exact details of how drugs are oxidized by the microsomal electron transport system are far from clear. A cyclic activity somewhat along the following lines is postulated (Gillette et al., 1972):

1) The substrate combines with the oxidized form of a haemoprotein called cytochrome P-450.

2) This oxidized complex is reduced by an electron from a flavoprotein, NADPH-cytochrome c reductase, to form a reduced substrate-cytochrome P-450 complex.

3) This combines with oxygen to form a substrate-cytochrome P-450-oxygen complex.

4) It is believed that a second electron then reduces this complex to form an active oxygen intermediate that decomposes, forming the product and oxidized cytochrome P-450.

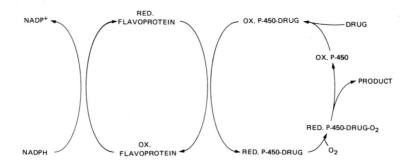

The exact composition of microsomal drug-metabolizing systems is uncertain. Cytochrome P-450 is closely bound to membranes and this hampers fractionation procedures. However, improved techniques involving solubilization and separation on DEAE-cellulose column chromatography have led to significant recent advances (Lu and Coon, 1968; Lu et al., 1972; Fujita and Mannering, 1973). The major components appear to be cytochrome P-450, NADPH-cytochrome c reductase and phospholipid. By re-combining these fractionated components, drug metabolizing systems can be formed. These reconstituted systems generally have similar properties to those of the microsomal preparations from which they are derived. Minor variations in procedure are critical and can alter the preference for one or other drug as substrate (Fujita and Mannering, 1973). However, with continued improvement in methodology, rapid advances can now be anticipated.

At least one other electron transport system is present in microsomes. This involves another cytochrome (cytochrome b_5), and another flavoprotein (NADH-cytochrome b_5 reductase). This system is more readily solubilized and is thought to be active in the desaturation of fatty acids (Oshino et al., 1971). It may play some part in microsomal drug metabolism. Indeed, a role for NADH as well as for NADPH was found in the first report of a microsomal drug metabolizing system (Mueller and Miller, 1949). Hildebrandt and Estabrook (1971) provided evidence that NADP can contribute to the reaction via cytochrome b_5, at least under certain circumstances. The latter is the only cytochrome other than cytochrome P-450 found in microsomes and could serve as a second electron donor for cytochrome P-450. However, during the induction of drug-metabolizing enzymes, there is only a delayed and slight increase in cytochrome

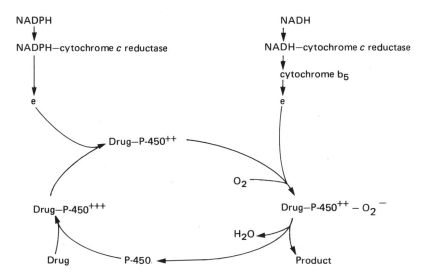

b_5. This contrasts with the prompt and marked increases in the components of the NADPH pathway of electron supply.

Microsomal drug metabolism involves reductive as well as oxidative reactions. Many azo dyes are cleaved reductively to primary aromatic amines. Nitro compounds such as chloramphenicol and nitrobenzene are reduced to primary amines. The studies of Hernandez et al. (1967) indicated that two mechanisms could account for microsomal reduction of azo dyes, (1) a carbon monoxide sensitive pathway involving cytochrome P-450 and destroyed by solubilization, and (2) a carbon monoxide insensitive pathway involving NADPH-cytochrome c reductase and not destroyed by solubilization. A mixed function oxidase that does not involve cytochrome P-450 has also been demonstrated in the N-oxidation of various N-alkyl-substituted amines (Ziegler et al., 1969). It is NADPH- and oxygen-dependent and acts on a number of secondary and tertiary amines, including tranquillizers, antihistamines, narcotics and ephedrine-like compounds.

3.4.2 Cytochrome P-450

Cytochrome P-450 is a phospholipid-protohaeme-sulphide-protein complex that owes its name to the fact that when exposed to carbon monoxide it absorbs light at 450nm. This property forms the basis of its analytical determination. It is the most abundant cytochrome of the liver and plays a major role in microsomal drug metabolism. As discussed by Mannering (1971), this latter conclusion is based on a number of observations:

1. Carbon monoxide combines with cytochrome P-450 and inhibits drug metabolism.
2. The inhibitory effect of carbon monoxide on microsomal drug metabolism is reversed by light with the maximum effect being obtained at a wavelength of 450nm. The latter corresponds to the peak absorption spectrum of cytochrome P-450 after exposure to carbon monoxide.
3. The conversion of cytochrome P-450 to its inactive form, cytochrome P-420, is associated with a corresponding reduction in drug-metabolizing activity.
4. Agents that raise or lower the level of microsomal cytochrome P-450 generally cause a corresponding rise or fall in the rate of microsomal drug metabolism.
5. Drugs that bind to cytochrome P-450 produce characteristic difference spectra. With some drugs there is a correlation between the kinetics of the binding and the kinetics of the metabolism of the same drugs.
6. Steroids are oxidized by both liver and adrenal cortex and both organs have a high microsomal content of cytochrome P-450.

Cytochrome P-450 is present in highest concentrations in the hepatic microsomes and in the adrenal cortical microsomes and mitochondria and in lesser quantities in the kidney and in the intestinal mucosa. Its hepatic concentration varies considerably from species to species, from strain to strain and even from individual to individual. Furthermore a number of endogenous and exogenous factors will influence the hepatic concentration at any one time (Mannering, 1971). Thus levels increase with advancing age in male, but not female, rats. Microsomal cytochrome P-450 is increased by fasting and is decreased by the administration of morphine and thyroxine. Some drugs such as phenobarbital which increase hepatic microsomal drug metabolism cause a parallel increase in microsomal cytochrome P-450. However, the rate of metabolism of some drugs is not increased when the microsomal level of cytochrome P-450 is elevated. The substrate specificities of microsomal enzyme systems involving cytochrome P-450 show marked differences between species. These may reflect differences in the form of cytochrome P-450 or in the way in which it is associated with the microsomal membrane.

3.4.3 Binding of Drugs to Cytochrome P-450

When the oxidized form of cytochrome P-450 combines with drugs and other substrates, it undergoes a conformational change which can be detected by spectrophotometry. This is done by observing the change in the difference spectrum. The latter is derived from the comparison of two cuvettes. A reference cuvette contains only microsomes and the experimental cuvette contains microsomes with the substrate or inhibitor. When the absorption spectrum of the reference cuvette is subtracted from the absorption spectrum of the experimental cuvette, two general types of difference spectra are produced, type I and modified type II (or reversed type I) (Remmer et al., 1966; Imai and Sato, 1966). Drugs giving these spectra have become known as type I and type II compounds respectively. Type I compounds produce a difference spectrum with an absorption maximum in the range of 385–390nm and an absorption minimum in the range of 419–425nm. Type II compounds produce almost the mirror image change with an absorption minimum at 390–405nm and an absorption maximum at 426-435nm (fig. 1). The addition of ethanol to microsomes produces a modified type II binding spectrum (Rubin et al., 1971).

Table IV gives the type of binding produced by a variety of drugs. It can be seen that the species and the pretreatment generally do not influence the type of binding spectrum produced. An exception is phenobarbital which gives a type I binding spectrum with rat hepatic microsomes and a type II spectrum with microsomes from rabbits. The basis of this difference is unknown. It is of interest that in one study (Jefcoate et al., 1969) type I binding was obtained with low concentrations of phenobarbital and type II binding with high concentrations.

The binding properties of cytochrome P-450 have also been found to vary with the age and sex of the animal and with the conditions of storage. Storage in the cold causes a loss of type I binding which may be the explanation for the loss of the microsomal drug metabolizing capacity for certain drugs. Loss of type I binding with drugs could be due to binding with endogenous substrates such as fatty acids released by lipid breakdown during storage. Type II binding is little affected by cold storage. It is well known that mature male rats metabolize some drugs faster than mature female rats but this sex difference is not seen in immature rats or in other laboratory animals. The basis of the difference appears to be an increased type I binding in mature male rats. The microsomal metabolism of type I drugs such as aminopyrine and hexobarbital are correspondingly increased (Schenkman et al., 1967). By contrast, there is no difference between the microsomes of mature male and female rats in their capacity to metabolize aniline or to combine with it to form a type II spectrum.

The view that drug binding is an essential step in the mechanism of drug hydroxylation has been strengthened by the apparent relationship between the

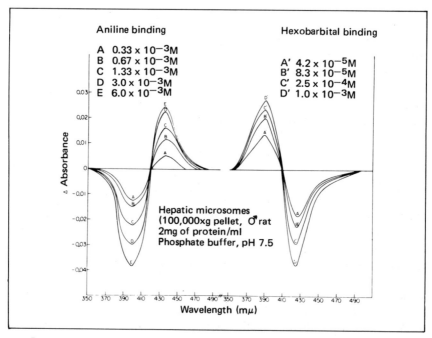

Fig. 1. Type I and type II binding spectra given by different concentrations of type I and type II compounds (hexobarbital and aniline respectively) (From Mannering, 1971).

Table IV. Qualitative differences in the binding of compounds to hepatic haemoprotein as determined by difference spectra (modified from Mannering, 1971)

Compound	Species	Pretreatment	Type of Binding	
			I	II
Acetanilide	Rat	—		+
Acetone	Rabbit	—		+
Alcoholic (methyl, ethyl, 2-propyl, iso-amyl)	Rabbit	Phenobarbital		+
Amines (n-propyl, n-pentyl, n-decyl, benzyl, cyclohexyl)	Rabbit	None		+
		Phenobarbital		+
p-Aminophenol	Rat	—		+
Aminopyrine	Rat	—	+	
Amylobarbital	Rat	—	+	
Amphetamine	Rat	—		+
Aniline	Rat	—		+
	Rat	Phenobarbital		+
	Rabbit	—		+
	Rabbit	Phenobarbital		+
3,4-Benzpyrene	Rat	3,4-Benzpyrene	+	
Chlorpromazine	Rat	—	+	
Cortisol	Rat	—		+
Coumarin	Rabbit	—	+	
Cyanide	Rat	—		+
Cyclohexane	Rat	—	+	
DDT	Rat	—	+	
Desdimethylimipramine	Mouse	Phenobarbital		+
Dioxane	Rabbit	Phenobarbital		+
β-Oestradiol	Rat	—	+	
Ethyl morphine	Rat, Rabbit	—		+
	Mouse, Guinea pig	—		
	Rat	Phenobarbital	+	
Hexobarbital	Rat, Rabbit	—	+	
	Rat, Mouse	Phenobarbital	+	
Imidazole	Mouse	—		+
Imipramine	Rat	—	+	
Metyrapone	Rat	Phenobarbital		+
	Mouse	Phenobarbital		+
Morphine	Rat	—	+	
Naphthalene	Mouse	Phenobarbital	+	
Nicotinamide	Rat, Mouse	—		+
	Rabbit	Phenobarbital		+
Nicotine	Rat	—		+
Phenacetin	Rabbit	—	+	
Phenobarbital (see text)	Rat	—	+	+
	Rabbit	—	+	+

Table IV. (continued)

Compound	Species	Pretreatment	Type of binding	
			I	II
Phenobarbital contd. (see text)	Rabbit	3-methyl-cholanthrene		+
	Rabbit	Phenobarbital		+
Progesterone	Rat	−	+	
Pyridine	Rat, Rabbit, Mouse	−		+
		−		+
	Rabbit	Phenobarbital		+
SKF 525-A	Rat, Mouse	−	+	
	Rat	Phenobarbital	+	
Testosterone	Rat	−	+	

kinetics of drug metabolism and the kinetics of drug binding. The dissociation constant (K_s) can be determined in much the same ways as the K_m (see section 4.1); i.e. by plotting the reciprocal of the drug concentration against the reciprocal of the altered optical density of the spectral change. In the case of a number of drugs, K_s and K_m for each compound were initially found to be similar. However, further studies have shown considerable discrepancy between K_s and K_m (Mannering, 1971). Even the absolute values for K_s and K_m have been found to vary between species and within the same species from one laboratory to another. These differences could partly reflect differences in the age or strain of animal used or in environmental conditions. The differences are perhaps not surprising when one considers the number of conditions that would have to be met for K_s to equal K_m (Mannering, 1971).

It should also be noted that the ability of compounds to form binding spectra with cytochrome P-450 does not automatically mean that they will be metabolized. For example, type II binding spectra are readily formed by many n-alkylamines but they are not metabolized. Conversely, microsomal hydroxylation can proceed without the development of binding spectra, as in the case of barbital and benzene.

3.4.4 Modified Forms of Cytochrome P-450 (Forms I, II, III; Cytochrome P-448)

Some drugs such as phenobarbital induce the metabolism of a much larger number of compounds than do the polycyclic hydrocarbons (such as 3-methylcholanthrene and 3,4-benzpyrene). Thus the mechanism for induction by phenobarbital could be different from that for the polycyclic hydrocarbons. Attempts to study the differences between the two inductive processes led to the conclusion that the polycyclic hydrocarbons cause the synthesis of a modified cytochrome P-450 (see Mannering, 1971). This was designated cytochrome P_1 - 450. However, it was soon found that after polycyclic hydrocarbon administration, the absorption maximum of reduced microsomal protein bound to CO was slightly different, i.e. at a wavelength of 448nm. Hence the term cytochrome P-448 was introduced. This compound does not form as a result of the combination of native cytochrome P-450 with polycyclic hydrocarbons (or their metabolites). Small amounts of cytochrome P-448 may be found in the microsomes of untreated animals. This would not be surprising when one considers that substances capable of inducing its synthesis may be present in the diets or atmosphere or could be produced by the intestinal flora. It is interesting to note in this regard that the earliest recognition of an exogenous inductive effect on drug metabolism was the finding that rancid diets contained steroids that stimulated the metabolism of aminoazo dyes.

The relative roles of cytochromes P-450 and P-448 in drug metabolism were studied by Jacobson et al. (1972) in a study that is also of interest in regard to the mechanisms of microsomal enzyme induction. Rats pretreated with phenobarbital or 3-methylcholanthrene developed increased hepatic microsomal levels of cytochrome P-450 and cytochrome P-448 respectively. In the former group, the anaesthetic effect of pentobarbital (30mg per kg) was abolished, whereas in the latter group pentobarbital anaesthesia was prolonged by 32 per cent. This prolongation of anaesthesia appeared to be due to a slower rate of pentobarbital metabolism because at the time of awakening from anaesthesia the brain levels of pentobarbital were the same as in control animals. These findings indicated that cytochrome P-448 might be less active than cytochrome P-450 in pentobarbital metabolism. This was supported by a study using the reconstituted hepatic microsomal system of Lu et al. (1972). The cytochrome P-448 fraction of this system supported pentobarbital metabolism at a rate of only 10 per cent of that supported by the cytochrome P-450 fraction.

Another interesting approach was that of Comai and Gaylor (1973) who reported the presence of three forms of cytochrome P-450, designated forms I, II and III. These are distinguished by visible spectral changes after binding with different ligands such as cyanide. The extent to which these spectral differences reflect structural changes in cytochrome P-450 is uncertain, and the relationship of these forms to cytochrome P-448 remains to be determined. Form III has the lowest affinity for cyanide, is inducible by 3-methylcholanthrene and may be identical with cytochrome P-448. Form II is preferentially induced by phenobarbital. Form I has the highest affinity for cyanide and is preferentially induced by ethanol, an observation first made by Joly et al. (1972).

4. Factors Affecting the Rate of Drug Metabolism

4.1 Enzyme Kinetics

Most drug biotransformations depend on enzymatic activity and therefore their velocities can be expressed in terms of two parameters that will be constant for any particular enzyme-substrate system. These are the maximum velocity (V) and the Michaelis constant (K_m). When the velocity is plotted against the substrate concentration (fig. 2) a rectangular hyperbola is obtained and the K_m represents the substrate concentration at the point of half maximum velocity ($\frac{V}{2}$). However, the maximum velocity can be difficult to determine experimentally and a convenient way of doing this is to use the well-known double reciprocal 'Lineweaver-Burk plot'. This involves the reciprocals of the velocity and the substrate concentration (fig. 3) and has the advantage that a straight line is obtained so that every point obtained experimentally contributes to the determination of V and K_m. Once these have been established for any particular enzyme system they can be employed to simplify experimental studies of that system in a number of ways. For example they can be used to distinguish it from other enzyme systems with similar substrate specificities. There are also therapeutic applications. For example, the K_m of alcohol dehydrogenase (ADH) is 2mM. Thus approximately doubling the K_m for ethanol will achieve almost full saturation of the ADH pathway. Thus in ethylene glycol poisoning (see section

7.1.1) where it is desirable to inhibit the metabolism of ethylene glycol by ADH, one can predict that an intake of ethanol sufficient to maintain a blood level of about 20mg per 100ml should be more than adequate. Higher doses of alcohol will be of no therapeutic benefit because the enzyme system will be already saturated and V will already have been reached.

4.2 Enzyme Control Mechanisms

Enzyme control mechanisms are of two major types, those that regulate the *activity* of each enzyme protein and those that regulate the *amount* of each enzyme protein. The former comprise a number of different mechanisms. Activation may occur as a result of structural modification. A prime example of this is the activation of many digestive enzymes which are secreted in inactive form from zymogen granules. Another example is 'molecular conversion', i.e. the

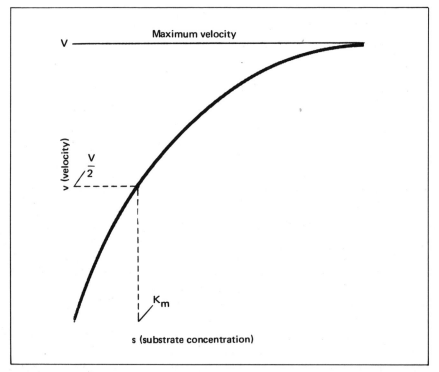

Fig. 2. Curve obtained by plotting the velocity of an enzyme reaction against the substrate concentration and showing the relationship between the half-maximum velocity ($\frac{V}{2}$) and the Michaelis constant (K_m). (From Loewy and Siekevitz, 1969).

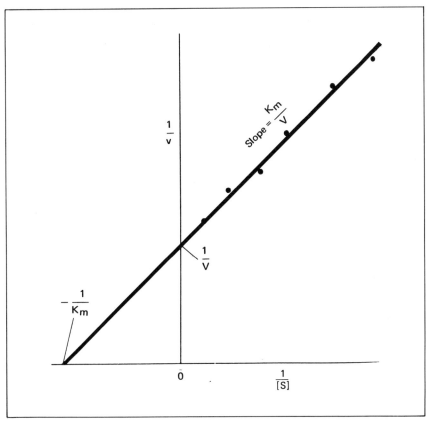

Fig. 3. The 'Lineweaver — Burk plot' of experimental values of v and [S] giving a straight line, which upon extrapolation, allows the determination of K_m and V. The advantage of a straight line is that each experimental point contributes to the determination of K_m and V. (From Loewy and Siekevitz, 1969).

association and dissociation of peptide subunits of the enzyme resulting in activation and inactivation respectively. For example, phosphorylase is inactivated when phosphate is removed from the enzyme by a phosphatase. Apparently this causes the enzyme to split into two inactive subunits. Phosphorylation reverses the process and produces activation.

Inhibition of the activity of an enzyme without a change in the amount of enzyme present is often produced by changes in the concentration of substrate or product. For example substrate inhibition of acetylcholinesterase can occur with high concentrations of acetylcholine. Product inhibition of hexokinase can occur with high levels of glucose-6-phosphate. The latter is an example of 'isosteric inhibition', that is, the inhibitor is a steric analogue of either the substrate or of the cofactor and therefore competes with either of them for the active site of the enzyme. Another type of enzyme activity modification is 'allosteric' activation or inhibition. In this type, the modifying compound is not sterically related to the substrate or to the cofactor. Therefore it does not compete for the active site of the enzyme, but acts at some other site. Feedback inhibition, in which an end product of a metabolic pathway inhibits an early step, is an example of this type of inhibition. For example isoleucine is synthesized at the end of a chain of four enzymatic steps. It inhibits the activity of the first step (the conversion of threonine to ketobutyrate) although it is not structurally similar to threonine.

The second major mechanism for the regulation of the activity of an enzyme involves a change in the amount of enzyme protein present. This may arise as a result of increased *de novo* synthesis (enzyme induction) or decreased degradation. Often enzyme induction is invoked to explain an increase in activity when strict evidence is not available of an increased rate of synthesis or even of an increased amount of enzyme. The rate of degradation can also be important. For example thymidine kinase and tryptophan pyrrolase are increased in activity by the administration of thymidine and tryptophan respectively. In both instances, the enhanced activity is the result of stabilization of the enzyme with a delayed rate of degradation. However, cortisol also stimulates the activity of tryptophan pyrrolase and this increase appears to be the result of enhanced enzyme synthesis.

4.3 Genetic Factors

Every clinician is aware of the striking individual variations in the responses of patients to a standard dose of a drug. Often these are due to environmental and pathological factors. However, there remain a high percentage where genetically determined factors are mainly responsible. The inherited variation is frequently due to a difference in the amount or activity of the relevant drug-metabolizing system. Therefore the condition is a type of inborn error of metabolism and a careful family study may reveal a high frequency amongst relatives (as is usually the case in the more florid inborn metabolic disturbances). In the preliminary investigation of an unusual therapeutic response to a standard dose of a drug, the comparison of its plasma levels to its pharmacological effects is essential. Thus in the case of an abnormally rapid metabolism of a drug, it might be found that clinical resistance was really due to failure to achieve adequate plasma levels. Conversely, where the rate of degradation is abnormally slow, plasma levels may reveal that the sensitivity to a drug is due to abnormally high concentrations after a standard dose.

Of course other genetically determined factors may play a role in unusual drug responses. These include variations in absorption, in plasma protein binding and in cell uptake, and may be specific for a particular drug or class of drugs. Furthermore, inherited metabolic disorders might produce disease states that could alter drug responses. For example, hypokalaemia due to renal tubular acidosis could predispose to digoxin toxicity. An inherited hepatic disorder could lower plasma protein levels generally and alter the transport and availability of drugs. A congenital haemoglobinopathy could make a patient more susceptible to drug-induced haemolysis or methaemoglobinaemia. Patients with sickle cell anaemia who receive anaesthetic agents may become hypoxic and this may lead to intravascular sickling and even infarction. Clearly, the numbers of ways in which genetic factors can influence drug responses are legion and the interested reader is referred to more detailed reviews (La Du, 1969; Vesell, 1969).

4.3.1 Inherited Variations in Drug-metabolizing Enzymes

Soon after the introduction of isoniazid (INH) for the treatment of tuberculosis, it became apparent that there were wide variations in the rates of INH metabolism. When the blood concentration of INH after a standard dose was studied in 267 individuals, it was found that there was bimodality of distribution (Evans et al., 1960). As can be seen from fig. 4, two subpopulations exist, designated as rapid inactivators and slow inactivators. The biological half-life of INH depends mainly on its rate of acetylation by hepatic N-acetyltransferase,

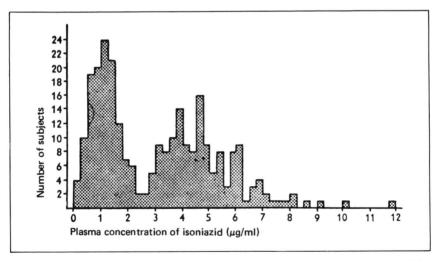

Fig. 4. Plasma concentrations of isoniazid 6 hours after each oral administration of the drug to 267 members of 53 families. (From Evans et al., 1960).

since acetyl-INH can be excreted more efficiently than INH. Family studies of fast and slow inactivators have shown that the rate of INH conjugation is determined by 2 autosomal genes at one locus; slow acetylators are homozygous for the recessive allele (rr), and fast acetylators are either RR or Rr. The two groups differ in the amounts of hepatic N-acetyltransferase present, but the enzyme appears to be qualitatively the same.

There is no apparent advantage in being a slow or fast inactivator of INH. Neither the outcome of the anti-tuberculous treatment nor the development of INH-resistant bacilli appears to be affected. Of course, slow acetylators are more prone to develop complications such as peripheral neuropathy, but this can be prevented by the administration of pyridoxine without impairing the therapy of the tuberculosis.

The recessive gene is so frequent that over half the population are slow acetylators. Thus a population survey in this situation was a practical means of study, especially as a simple method was used, namely a single blood assay after a standard oral dose. However, in many other pharmacogenetic studies, population surveys are inefficient, usually because the abnormal gene is present in only a small percentage of the population or because the methodology is cumbersome and expensive for large surveys. The above study by Evans and his associates also highlights the importance of carefully selecting the conditions of study in advance. It has been estimated that if the blood samples had been collected at 2 hours rather than at 6 hours, a continuous, unimodal curve would have been obtained.

A number of other drugs are acetylated by hepatic N-acetyltransferase. These include sulphamethazine, hydrallazine (Apresoline), diaminodiphenyl-sulphone (Dapsone), phenelzine (Nardil), sulphafurazole (Gantrisin) and sulpha-diazine. Polymorphism of N-acetyltransferase activity appears to be of little clinical significance for the latter two drugs, but studies of sulphamethazine clearance show a clearly bimodal distribution and this drug is sometimes used to type fast and slow acetylators.

Succinylcholine sensitivity is another example of an inherited variation in drug-metabolizing enzymes. An occasional patient given this muscle relaxant will remain paralyzed for much longer than expected and may require artificial respiration for hours. However, in contrast to the slow excretors of INH, sensitivity to succinylcholine appears to be due to a qualitative rather than a quantitative difference in enzyme activity. The enzyme responsible is cholinesterase present in the serum. A number of atypical cholinesterases, with a low affinity for choline-esters, have been found in susceptible individuals. Spectrophotometric methods to distinguish these different types are now available. An even rarer type of cholinesterase abnormality is associated with an increased serum concentration of the enzyme. Affected individuals are resistant, rather than sensitive, to the drug.

4.3.2 Inherited Metabolic Disorders that Modify Drug Toxicity

An example of this is glucose-6-phosphate dehydrogenase (G6PD) deficiency which is a common cause of drug-sensitive haemolysis. This is transmitted by a gene on the X chromosome, giving a sex-linked inheritance. It is common amongst negroes and Southern Europeans; 15 per cent of negro males and 1.6 per cent of negro females in the United States are affected. The reduced level of G6PD in the red cell impairs the formation of NADPH which is the reduced cofactor for glutathione reductase and consequently glutathione levels are reduced. The supply of glutathione appears to be critical for maintaining the red cell membrane. Its level falls when the red cells of G6PD-deficient individuals are incubated with certain drugs. A large number of drugs is capable of producing haemolysis in these people. These include primaquine, quinidine, chloroquine, nitrofurantoin (Furadantin), naphthalene, various sulphonamides, sulphones, phenacetin, salicylates and probenecid (Benemid).

4.3.3 Inherited Deficiency of Drug-activating Enzymes

Some drugs are inactive until metabolized *in vivo* by specific enzyme systems. One group of drugs exemplifying this includes such purine antimetabolites as azathioprine, 6-mercaptopurine, 6-thioguanine and 8-azaguanine. Their activation is catalyzed by the hepatic enzyme hypoxanthine-guanine phosphoribosyltransferase (H-G-PRT) (Kelly et al., 1969). Rare cases of gout (including the Lesch-Nyhan syndrome) are due to an inherited deficiency of this enzyme. Feedback inhibition of purine synthesis is impaired (fig. 5). Because H-G-PRT is also needed for the activation of purine antimetabolites, the usual antineoplastic effect of these drugs is reduced. A similar inhibition may appear in severe hepatic disease of any cause.

Patients with H-G-PRT deficiency also have an impaired response to allopurinol, a drug widely used in the treatment of gout. Allopurinol acts in two ways (Seegmiller et al., 1967). First, it is a direct inhibitor of xanthine oxidase; uric acid formation is thus reduced at the expense of increased levels of xanthine and hypoxanthine. These latter compounds are more soluble than uric acid and are excreted in the urine with apparently little risk of calculus formation. This effect of allopurinol is independent of H-G-PRT activity. The second effect depends on the activation of allopurinol by H-G-PRT to form a compound that acts as a 'feedback inhibitor' of purine synthesis.

4.3.4 Inherited Resistance to Coumarin Anticoagulants

An inherited form of coumarin resistance has been reported by O'Reilly (1970). The condition is rare and is inherited as an autosomal Mendelian domin-

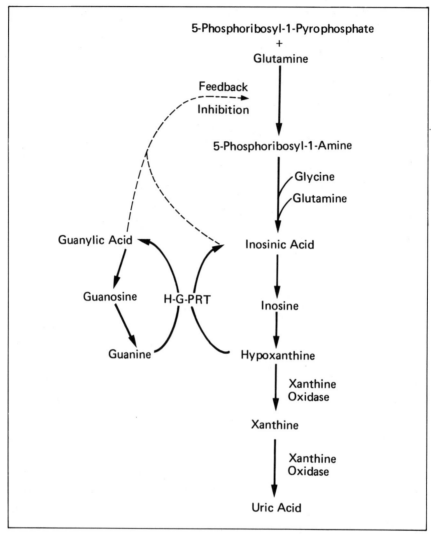

Fig. 5. Pathway of purine catabolism showing the role of H-G-PRT in feedback inhibition of uric acid synthesis.

ant. Approximately 20 times the usual dose of warfarin is required to achieve a therapeutic response and there is a comparable resistance to the antidotal effects of vitamin K. It is thought that an enzyme or a receptor site involved in the synthesis of the clotting factors II, VII, IX and X may have been modified by genetic mutation in some way to alter its affinity for both coumarin anticoagulants and vitamin K.

4.4 Microsomal Enzyme Induction

4.4.1 Introduction

There are many drugs whose administration stimulates not only their own biotransformation but that of a variety of other agents as well. This effect seems to be mainly due to an increased synthesis of microsomal drug-metabolizing enzymes in the liver and is commonly referred to as 'enzyme induction'. It has been the subject of many reviews (Gillette, 1963; Conney, 1967, 1971; Gelboin, 1971; Remmer, 1972) and only the main points will be covered here.

Most of the enzyme activities that are enhanced by drug pretreatment are localized in the microsomal fraction. Although a large number of chemically unrelated compounds may induce the same enzyme system, some enzymes will be induced by one class of compound and not by another. For example, microsomal androgen hydroxylase activity is stimulated by pretreatment with phenobarbital but not with 3,4-benzpyrene. By contrast, the hydroxylation of 3,4-benzpyrene is enhanced by pretreatment with the substrate itself or with phenobarbital. Thus the profile of enzyme systems that can be activated will vary from one inducing agent to another.

Of course, some of the substrates for these enzymes are endogenous compounds such as steroids and thus microsomal enzyme induction is of potential physiological importance. However, the main interest in microsomal enzyme induction has centred around its pharmacological effects. The therapeutic effects of drugs and their side effects may be significantly enhanced or inhibited depending on whether the active agents responsible are the ingested drugs themselves or some metabolites.

The first report of a stimulatory effect of a foreign compound on hepatic microsomal enzymes was made by Brown et al. in 1954 in the course of a study of dietary factors on hepatic N-demethylase activity. Since that time, some hundreds of drugs, insecticides, carcinogens and other compounds have been shown to be capable of stimulating hepatic microsomal drug-metabolizing enzymes (Conney, 1969, 1971; Mannering, 1968). Examples of these are shown in table V. Most commonly used classes of drugs have been shown to be involved. In addition, environmental exposure to chemicals is a potential source of stimulation of microsomal enzymes although one can only guess at its significance in modern society. Examples of such chemicals include polycyclic aromatic hydrocarbons (in cigarette smoke, polluted city air and barbecued foods), halogenated hydrocarbon insecticides, urea herbicides, food preservatives, dyes used as colouring agents and caffeine in foodstuffs. Materials used in the bedding of laboratory animals (for example, cedar chips) are also known to stimulate hepatic drug metabolism. The importance of insecticides was first noticed when studies on drug metabolism were disrupted for weeks following the spraying of

Table V. Compounds studied as potential stimulators of drug metabolism (Conney, 1967)

Pharmacological action	Drug tested	Effect
Hypnotics and sedatives	Barbiturates	+
	Glutethimide (Doriden)	+
	Chlorobutanol (Chloretone)	+
	Urethane	+
	Carbromal (Adalin)	+
	Pyridione (Persedon)	+
	Methyprylone (Noludar)	+
	Ethanol	±
	Chloral hydrate	±
	Ethinamate (Valmid)	0
	Hydroxydione (Viadril)	0
	Thalidomide	0
	Paraldehyde	0
Anaesthetic gases	Nitrous oxide	+
	Methoxyflurane	+
	Halothane	±
	Ether	±
Central nervous system stimulators	Nikethamide (Coramine)	+
	Bemegride	+
	Pentylenetetrazol (Metrazol)	0
	Amphetamine	0
Anticonvulsants	Methylphenylethylhydantoin (Mesantoin)	+
	Diphenylhydantoin (Dilantin)	+
	Paramethadione (Paradione)	+
	Trimethadione (Tridione)	0
Tranquillizers	Phenaglycodol (Ultran)	+
	Meprobamate	+
	Chlordiazepoxide (Librium)	+
Antipsychotics	Chlorpromazine	+
	Triflupromazine	+
	Promazine	+
Hypoglycaemic agents and related sulphonamides	Tolbutamide (Orinase)	+
	Carbutamide	+
	Sulphaethidole	0
	Sulphanilamide	0
Anti-inflammatory agents	Phenylbutazone	+

Table V. (continued)

Pharmacological action	Drug tested	Effect
Muscle relaxants	Orphenadrine	+
	Carisoprodol	+
	Zoxazolamine	±
Analgesics	Aminopyrine	+
	Aspirin	0
	Morphine and Levorphan	Decrease
Antihistaminics	Chlorcyclizine	+
	Diphenhydramine	+
Alkaloids	Nicotine	+
	Cotinine	+
Insecticides	DDT	+
	Dieldrin	+
	Aldrin	+
	Pyrethrums	0
Steroid hormones	4-Androstene-3,17-dione	+
and related substances	Testosterone	+
	4-Chlorotestosterone	+
	19-Nortestosterone	+
	Methyltestosterone	+
	4-Chloro-19-nortestosterone acetate	+
	4-Chloro-17a-methyl-19-nortestosterone	+
	17a-ethyl-19-nortestosterone (Norethandrolone)	+
	Cortisone	+
	Prednisolone	+
	Norethynodrel	+
	Progesterone	±
	Estradiol	Decrease
	Cholesterol	0
	Oxidized cholesterol	+
	Oxidized dihydrocholesterol	+
	Oxidized ergosterol	+
Carcinogenic polycyclic aromatic hydrocarbons	3-Methylcholanthrene,3,4-benz-pyrene, 1,2,5,6-dibenzanthracene	+

animal quarters with chlordane (Hart and Fouts, 1965). Other insecticides found to stimulate microsomal enzymes include DDT, DDE, methoxychlor, aldrin, endrin, dieldrin, heptachlor and benzene hexachloride. Their effects commonly last for several weeks, even up to three months in some cases, after a single exposure. The amount of DDT required to affect hepatic microsomal enzyme activity is extremely small. As little as $10\mu g$ of DDT per gram of fat in the rat is associated with enhanced pentobarbital metabolism. Many people have comparable concentrations of DDT and other insecticides in their fat so that it is possible that their rate of metabolism of some drugs could be increased. The potential importance of this is all the more when one considers the very slow rate of elimination of DDT from the body. Kolmodin et al. (1969) found that pesticide factory workers exposed to DDT and lindane had an enhanced rate of metabolism of antipyrine. It is reasonable to expect that their metabolism of a number of other drugs would also have been increased. In contrast to the halogenated hydrocarbons, organophosphorus insecticides, when given chronically, inhibit the microsomal hydroxylation of drugs and steroids.

4.4.2 Membrane and Phospholipid Changes

Hepatic size is commonly increased by drug pretreatment. Many polycyclic hydrocarbons increase the amount of hepatic protein, but not its concentration. By contrast, phenobarbital and many other drugs increase both the amount and concentration of hepatic protein. Part of this is due to an increased microsomal mass. Hepatic microsomal protein (expressed per gm of wet liver) increases by some 20–40% after phenobarbital administration. The increase is greater in the agranular portion of the microsomal fraction, in keeping with electron microscopic observations of proliferation of the SER. Orrhenius and Ernster (1964) found that 6 hours after a single injection of phenobarbital given to rabbits, the first changes were enhanced levels of aminopyrine demethylase, NADPH-cytochrome c reductase, and cytochrome P-450 in the rough-surfaced vesicle fraction. Between 6 and 12 hours, the increases began to taper off in the rough vesicle fraction while a progressive rise in enzyme levels began in the smooth vesicle fraction. Repeated doses of phenobarbital produced increases in both rough and smooth-surfaced membranes of the endoplasmic reticulum but the latter effect was the most marked and was associated with marked enhancement of the activities of drug-metabolizing enzymes (Remmer and Merker, 1963; Orrhenius and Ernster, 1964). These observations have since been confirmed in many laboratories and many other drugs have been found to produce similar effects. However, some drugs (such as 3-methylcholanthrene and 3,4-benzpyrene) stimulate microsomal drug metabolism without producing any significant proliferation of the SER (Fouts and Rogers, 1965).

Hepatic microsomal phospholipid is generally increased during enzyme induction. Indeed a number of studies have shown a sometimes close but poorly understood correlation between microsomal drug metabolism and microsomal phospholipid content. The elevation of the latter during enzyme induction has been shown to involve phosphatidylcholine, phosphatidylethanolamine and lyso-phosphatidylcholine (Orrhenius et al., 1965; Cooper and Feuer, 1973). By contrast, the administration of a hepatotoxin such as CCl_4 is associated with a reduced activity of drug-metabolizing enzymes and a lower content of phospholipid (Cooper and Feuer, 1973). The latter authors also showed that choline deficiency in rats altered the effects of foreign compounds on both the phospholipid composition and enzyme activity of hepatic microsomes. Choline deficiency alone caused a decrease of drug-metabolizing activity and lowered all phospholipid fractions except phosphatidic acid. Choline deficiency also antagonized the rise in microsomal phospholipid content and the induction of drug metabolism produced by the administration of phenobarbital or of 4-methyl-coumarin. Conversely, the fall in phospholipid and the inhibition of drug metabolism produced by CCl_4 were both comparably reduced by choline deficiency.

However, the correlation between the phospholipid content and the drug-metabolizing activity of hepatic microsomes is by no means constant. Thus Orrhenius and Ericsson (1966) found that an inducing course of phenobarbital given to rats maintained a high microsomal phospholipid content for 15 days, whereas aminopyrine demethylase activity returned to normal within 5 days. A second course of phenobarbital was given when the enzyme activity was back to normal and when the phospholipid content was still raised. This resulted in a slower increase in aminopyrine demethylase activity than with the initial course.

4.4.3 Mechanisms of Enzyme Induction (see also section 3.4.4)

The molecular basis for hepatic microsomal enzyme induction by structurally unrelated foreign compounds is unknown. Some of the possible mechanisms that could be considered are:

1) Interaction with DNA to stimulate the synthesis of specific messenger RNA;

2) Interaction with repressors synthesized by a regulator gene or with other regulators of gene function, such as histones;

3) Interaction with the endoplasmic reticulum to enhance the translation of messenger RNA on the ribosomes;

4) Interaction with the enzyme itself to inhibit its degradation or to prevent feedback inhibition of its synthesis;

5) Stimulation of production of a specific protein that activates an inactive form of the enzyme.

The increased microsomal drug-metabolizing activity after drug pretreatment is not due to the presence of the drug itself. The direct addition of phenobarbital and other inducing agents to hepatic homogenates does not stimulate drug metabolism. In fact, it is of interest that nearly all drugs that act as inducers are lipid-soluble and capable of penetrating the microsomes and of exerting a biphasic effect on drug metabolism. Thus the initial effect of an inducing agent (for approximately the first six hours) is inhibition of enzyme activity. This is apparently due to competition for binding to cytochrome P-450. There then follows a progressive rise in activity (usually after 12 hours) as enzyme induction develops.

Attempts to show that drugs increase drug-metabolizing activity by increasing the concentration of a possible endogenous activator or cofactor, or by decreasing the level of an inhibitor, have been unsuccessful (Conney, 1967). Liver homogenate from animals treated with phenobarbital or 3-methylcholanthrene does not alter the activity of drug-metabolizing enzymes in control liver homogenate when the two homogenates are mixed.

Hormonal influences appear to play little part in microsomal enzyme induction despite their importance in microsomal drug metabolism generally (see section 4.5). Thus phenobarbital and 3-methylcholanthrene enhance the activities of various drug-metabolizing enzyme systems in rats even after hypophysectomy, adrenalectomy, castration, oophorectomy or thyroidectomy (Conney, 1967). Furthermore, microsomal enzymes can be induced in hepatic cells in tissue culture (Gielen and Nebert, 1971).

The possibility of enhanced rates of synthesis of microsomal enzymes is raised by the observations of increased concentrations of microsomal protein after pretreatment with some inducing agents. Enhanced microsomal protein and haeme synthesis is apparent within 3—5 hours of phenobarbital administration (Remmer, 1972). The first enzyme to be induced is actually mitochondrial, namely δ-ALA-synthetase. Haeme synthesis rises steadily for 16 hours, then levels off for two days, then starts to decline. Studies using C^{14} leucine have shown pronounced increases in the incorporation of the tracer into microsomal proteins after pretreatment with various drugs. The effect begins within 15 minutes of 3-methylcholanthrene administration. The effect of phenobarbital on microsomal NADPH-cytochrome c reductase was studied by Kuriyama et al. (1969). There was a prompt increase in the rate of synthesis and the induced enzyme was chromatographically and immunochemically identical to the normal hepatic enzyme. However, part of the rise in the amount of the reductase was due to a concomitant decrease in the rate of degradation. Thus decreased breakdown of microsomal enzymes appears to play some part in the enhanced enzyme activity produced by drugs. Similarly, phospholipid catabolism may also be impaired by drug pretreatment (Holtzman and Gillette, 1968).

However, the major factor in enzyme induction appears to be enhanced enzyme synthesis. Support for this is derived from the observations that inhibitors of protein synthesis or of DNA-dependent RNA synthesis prevent the induction of drug-metabolizing enzymes (see Gelboin, 1971). Thus induction by 3-methylcholanthrene or by phenobarbital is blocked by ethionine, puromycin, or actinomycin D. These inhibitors block protein synthesis by different mechanisms.

Ethionine is the ethyl analogue of methionine. Its effect is due to its incorporation into S-adenosyl-ethionine, thus preventing the formation of S-adenosyl-methionine and inhibiting the synthesis of ATP. This effect is reversed by methionine administration. The effects of ATP depletion on protein synthesis are complex and may occur at many different levels. Puromycin blocks microsomal protein synthesis by preventing the transfer of soluble RNA-bound aminoacid into polypeptide chains. When given alone, it has no acute effect on drug-metabolizing enzymes. However, induction by phenobarbital is completely blocked.

Actinomycin D binds to DNA, and inhibits protein synthesis by preventing the DNA-directed synthesis of nuclear RNA. It effectively abolishes the induction of a variety of enzymes by phenobarbital and 3-methylcholanthrene. Like puromycin and ethionine, it blocks the induction of azo dye reductase by 3-methylcholanthrene. However, the induction of this reductase by phenobarbital is blocked by puromycin or by ethionine, but not by actinomycin D. This suggests that induction of this enzyme might involve different mechanisms.

From a review of studies in cell cultures, Gelboin (1971) has suggested the following sequence of events in microsomal enzyme induction:

1) RNA synthesis. Upon addition to the culture medium the inducing agent is incorporated into the cell within several minutes. There follows a rapid interaction between inducer and receptor site leading to a period of early RNA synthesis. This stage is inhibited by actinomycin D. It is independent of translation since it occurs in the presence of other inhibitors of enzyme synthesis.

2) Protein synthesis. This stage seems to involve the polymerization of aminoacid into polypeptide chains. It is sensitive to other inhibitors of protein synthesis, but can proceed in the absence of the RNA synthesis stage and is therefore not inhibited by actinomycin D.

3) Assembly of newly formed polypeptide chains. This is independent of the second stage and may persist for up to two hours.

The specific protein assembled in the microsomes during the induction process may be the enzyme itself or a protein capable of activating the enzyme by an allosteric mechanism. All of these events appear before there are gross changes in either protein or in RNA synthesis. This suggests that the RNA and protein involved in the induction of enzymes are very small percentages of total cell RNA and protein. Thus, many of the gross changes of RNA and protein synthesis may be subsequent to, and parallel, but may not be directly responsible for the appearance of the early increases in enzyme levels.

4.4.4 Effects of Species, Strain and Age on Enzyme Induction

The administration of well known inducing agents such as phenobarbital produce a generalised increase in the activities of hepatic microsomal drug-metabolizing enzymes within a wide range of experimental conditions. However, there are abundant examples of the fact that extrapolation of data from one experimental situation to another is fraught with pitfalls (Conney, 1967). Dietary factors, such as choline deficiency and the presence of hepatotoxins (see section 4.4.2) may modify the response. Species differences may be important. Thus DDT stimulates drug metabolism in the rat, but not in the mouse. It also decreases the storage of dieldrin (apparently by accelerating its metabolism) in the rat, swine and sheep, but not in the chicken. In the rat, phenylbutazone stimulates the 6β-, 7α-, and 16α-hydroxylation of testosterone, whereas in the dog, only 6β-, and 16α-hydroxylation are stimulated.

Even within a given species there may be genetically determined differences. In one study, phenobarbital caused large increases in the hepatic metabolism of hexobarbital in the cotton-tail rabbit, but produced very little change in the English rabbit; similarly, benzpyrene hydroxylation was stimulated by phenobarbital in only two out of six strains of rabbit studied (Gram et al., 1965). Such genetically determined variations might account for some of the occasional failures of enzyme induction in laboratory animals. These have their human counterparts. For example, the anticoagulant effect of bishydroxycoumarin is reduced in most people by phenobarbital, but an occasional subject will show no such response to the barbiturate.

Age will also affect the response of hepatic microsomes to an inducing agent. Newborn animals have very little ability to metabolize drugs such as hexobarbital, aminopyrine, phenacetin, amphetamine and chlorpromazine. Newborn mice treated with 10mg of hexobarbital per kg sleep for longer than 6 hours, whereas adult mice treated with 10 times this dose regain righting reflexes in less than 1 hour. However, the administration of drugs such as phenobarbital or chlordane to newborn rabbits increases hepatic drug metabolism. A similar enhancement may be produced by giving the drugs to the pregnant rabbits (in the last 4 days of foetal life) or to lactating rabbits. In the latter case, the phenobarbital produces its inducing effects in the nurslings without producing sedation. Generally speaking, 'inducing agents' produce a greater increase in hepatic drug metabolism in immature male and in adult female rats than in adult male rats. However, this may merely reflect the fact that the adult male rat normally has a higher level of drug-metabolizing enzymes.

4.4.5 Enzyme Induction in Extrahepatic Tissues

Low levels of drug-metabolizing enzymes are found in extrahepatic tissues, particularly the lung, gastro-intestinal tract and the kidney. Using very sensitive fluorometric and histochemical techniques, it has been shown that the administration of polycyclic hydrocarbons increases the activity of benzpyrene hydroxylase in the kidney, small intestine, placenta, skin and ovaries, and causes the appearance of activity, previously too low to be detected, in the thyroid, lung and testis of rats (Wattenberg and Leong, 1962; Wattenberg et al., 1962; Conney, 1971). In the gastro-intestinal tract, dietary factors may play a role. Starvation alone for 72 hours causes a 15-fold rise in rat duodenal benzpyrene hydroxylase activity (Wattenberg et al., 1962). Several phenothiazine derivatives increase the activities of this enzyme in the gastro-intestinal tract, kidney, lung, spleen and thymus (Wattenberg and Leong, 1965). However, the administration of phenobarbital to the rat has no effect on gastro-intestinal or placental benzpyrene hydroxylase, and does not increase the activity of pentobarbital oxidase in lung, nitroreductase in kidney, or aminopyrine demethylase in kidney, heart, spleen, brain, muscle or lung. In contrast to the above findings in rats, phenobarbital administration to rabbits increases the activities of drug-metabolizing enzymes in the kidneys (Uehleke and Greim, 1968). Others have demonstrated the presence of inducible N-demethylase, hydroxylase, reductase and glucuronyl transferase in non-hepatic tissues (see Conney, 1971). These findings suggest that these enzymes may play some part in the biotransformation of drugs and other foreign compounds. It is also conceivable that inducible drug-metabolizing enzymes in the gastro-intestinal tract may influence the rates of drug absorption, although this aspect of enzyme induction appears to have received little attention.

4.4.6 Enzyme Induction in Humans

Allowing for variations between species, the response of microsomal enzyme systems in humans to foreign compounds is much the same as that seen in laboratory animals. Examples of enzyme induction in humans are shown in table VI. As discussed elsewhere (see sections 4.4.10, 7.2) this could be of therapeutic importance in a number of clinical situations, notably in anticoagulant therapy, in the treatment of epilepsy and in the treatment of alcoholics. For example, the administration to epileptic patients of diphenylhydantoin with phenobarbital results in significantly lower plasma levels of diphenylhydantoin than when this agent is given alone. Fortunately, this does not give rise to clinically apparent problems because phenobarbital also has anticonvulsant properties. However, it is possible that the simultaneous administration of

Table VI. Enzyme induction in humans

Inducing agent	Enhanced metabolism
Phenobarbital and other barbiturates	Bilirubin (Crigler and Gold, 1969) Cortisol (Burstein and Klaiber, 1965) Coumarin anticoagulants (MacDonald, Robinson, Sylwester and Jaffe, 1969) Digitoxin (Jeliffe and Blankenhorn, 1961) Diphenylhydantoin (Cucinell, Conney, Sansur and Burns, 1965) Dipyrone (Remmer, 1962)
Glutethimide	Dipyrone (Remmer, 1962) Warfarin (MacDonald, Robinson, Sylwester and Jaffe, 1969)
Phenylbutazone	Aminopyrine (Chen, Vrindten, Dayton and Burns, 1962) Cortisol (Kuntzman, Jacobson and Conney, 1966)
Ethanol	Aminopyrine (Vesell, Page and Passananti, 1971) CCl_4 (Hasumura, Teschke and Lieber, 1974) Hexobarbital (Mallov and Baesl, 1972) Meprobamate (Misra, Lefèvre, Ishii, Rubin and Lieber, 1971) Pentobarbital (Rubin and Lieber, 1968; Misra et al., 1971) Tolbutamide (Carulli, Manenti and Gallo, 1971) Zoxazolamine (Mallov and Baesl, 1972)
Chloral hydrate	Bishydroxycoumarin (Cucinell, Conney, Sansur and Burns, 1965)
Meprobamate	Meprobamate (Douglas, Ludwig and Smith, 1963)
Diphenylhydantoin	Cortisol (Werk, MacGee and Sholiton, 1964)
o,p´-DDD	Cortisol (Bledsoe, Island, Ney and Liddle, 1964)
DDT, Lindane	Antipyrine (Kolmodin, Azarnoff and Sjoqvist, 1969)
Cigarette smoke	3,4-Benzpyrene (Welch, Harrison, Gommi, Poppers, Finster and Conney, 1969) Nicotine (Beckett and Triggs, 1967)

diphenylhydantoin with other drugs that stimulate its metabolism, but are not themselves anticonvulsants, could impair the degree of control of the epilepsy in these patients. This metabolic tolerance could also contribute significantly to the enhanced tolerance to sedatives and anaesthetic agents that is seen in patients on prolonged anticonvulsant therapy and in drug addicts and alcoholics. It might conceivably play a role in carcinogenesis. It is important to bear in mind that induction may result from environmental and occupational exposure to foreign compounds in people receiving no therapeutic agents (see section 4.4.1).

4.4.7 Physiological Implications of Enzyme Induction

Microsomal enzymes act on endogenous as well as on exogenous substrates. Hence the increased drug-metabolizing potential of drug-treated animals is of potential physiological importance for the whole organism. However, there have been relatively few studies into this aspect of drug induction. Those that have been carried out have been mainly in animals and their relevance to human physiology is uncertain.

The best known endogenous substrates of microsomal hydroxylases are the steroids. The treatment of rats with a standard 'inducing course' of pheno-barbital enhances the hydroxylation of androgens, oestrogens, progestational steroids and adrenocortical steroids. Steroid hydroxylase activity can be induced by a number of structurally unrelated foreign compounds including pheno-barbital, diphenylhydantoin, chlorcyclizine, orphenadrine, phenylbutazone, chlordane, DDT and oρ'-DDD. These changes in enzyme metabolism are reflected in changes in the physiological responses to injected steroids in animals (Conney, 1971). Thus phenobarbital pretreatment inhibits the growth promoting effect of testosterone on the seminal vesicles of immature male rats. It also inhibits the action of oestradiol, oestrone and stilboestrol on the rat uterus. The uterotropic action of mestranol and other oral contraceptive agents in rats is also impaired by treatment with phenobarbitone.

Rats treated with barbiturates develop hypertrophy of the thyroid gland (Owen et al., 1971) and changes in thyroxine metabolism (Oppenheimer et al., 1968). The latter group postulated the following sequence of events. The administration of phenobarbital causes a primary increase in hepatocellular binding, as a result of both increased liver mass and increased binding per gm of liver. The ensuing shift of thyroxine from non-hepatic hormonal stores to the liver increases the pool of exchangeable hepatic thyroxine. This stimulates hepatic deiodinative and excretory processes and increases the deiodinative and faecal clearances of thyroxine. The fall in plasma and in non-hepatic thyroxine stimulates thyroidal secretion. A new steady state is achieved in which plasma and non-hepatic thyroxine stores have returned to near normal.

Calcium and folate metabolism can also be disturbed by hepatic enzyme induction (Latham et al., 1973). An English survey showed that epileptic patients frequently had biochemical evidence of osteomalacia and that this was related to the administration of anticonvulsant drugs. This now appears to be due to the induction of enzymes responsible for the metabolism of vitamin D. Anticonvulsant drugs producing this derangement of calcium metabolism can be listed in the following order of decreasing importance: pheneturide (Benuride), primidone (Mysoline), phenytoin (Epanutin), and phenobarbitone. Latham et al. (1973) showed that the enzyme-inducing properties of these drugs were of approximately the same order. Serum folate levels are also reduced during anti-convulsant therapy and impaired absorption may play some part in this. However, these drugs also induce hepatic enzymes involved in folate metabolism and this may contribute to the folate deficiency of epileptics (see also section 7.2.2).

As discussed in section 6.10, microsomal drug oxidations are inefficient because they are not linked to ATP synthesis and therefore their induction could lead to wastage of calories. Bilirubin metabolism is also affected by various inducing agents. Barbiturates given to animals enhance the microsomal glucur-onidation of bilirubin, stimulate bile flow and accelerate the *in vivo* metabolism of bilirubin (see section 4.4.10). Agents capable of inducing microsomal enzymes have also been implicated in the suppression of the immune response (Park and Brody, 1971) and in alteration of hepatic blood flow (Ohnhaus et al., 1971).

4.4.8 Effect of Enzyme Induction on Duration of Drug Action

The administration of drugs that induce hepatic microsomal enzymes generally decreases the pharmacological effectiveness of a variety of therapeutic agents that are metabolized in the SER. These include such well known agents as phenobarbital, hexobarbital, diphenylhydantoin, zoxazolamine, meprobamate and chlorpromazine. The resulting decreased effectiveness of a standard dose of these drugs is often referred to as an increase in metabolic tolerance.

The speed with which enzyme induction can be achieved and the length of time for which it remains varies considerably. Age, sex, species and other conditions are relevant, but the major variation is with the drugs used to induce microsomal enzymes and the drugs used to test enzyme induction. For example, zoxazolamine is a muscle relaxant that is hydroxylated by hepatic microsomes to an inactive metabolite. The administration of 3,4-benzpyrene results in a maximum shortening of the effect of a standard dose of zoxazolamine within 24 hours. By contrast, phenobarbital administration has to be continued for some 3–4 days before the maximum reduction in the effect of zoxazolamine is achieved. The duration of paralysis after the relaxant in one study was 17 minutes after 3,4-benzpyrene pretreatment, 102 minutes after phenobarbital pretreatment, but over 11 hours in control rats (Conney, 1967). That this is an example of metabolic tolerance is shown by the fact that the biological half life of zoxazolamine in the corresponding three groups of animals was 10 minutes, 48 minutes and 9 hours.

4.4.9 Effect of Enzyme Induction on Drug Complications

The toxic effects of any drug may be either decreased or increased as a result of induction of hepatic microsomal enzymes. The direction of the change will depend on whether the toxic effects are due to the administered agent or to one of its metabolites. Examples of the former are zoxazolamine, meprobamate, pentobarbital, strychnine and oral anticoagulants. Thus in one study all of the control rats were killed by a dose of 150mg/kg of zoxazolamine whereas no rats died when the same treatment was preceded by a single injection of 3-methylcholanthrene (Conney, 1967). This sparing effect of an inducing agent can actually be dangerous in some clinical situations. A classical example of this is the patient on oral anticoagulant therapy whose prothrombin time is stabilised at a time when he is receiving some other agent that is capable of inducing microsomal enzymes. Sudden cessation of the inducing agent will produce a decrease in the required dose of the anticoagulant. However, this will usually pass unsuspected until the patient next has a check of the prothrombin time or actually starts to bleed.

Examples of agents whose toxicity is enhanced by enzyme induction are the insecticides Schradan and Guthion (Conney, 1971). These are metabolized by hepatic microsomes to cholinesterase inhibitors. Control animals treated with Schradan have a mortality of 6% whereas after pretreatment with a barbiturate, the mortality rises to 75%. Similarly the lethality of Guthion is increased by pretreatment with 3-methylcholanthrene but decreased by pretreatment with the enzyme inhibitor SKF 525-A. The toxicity of carbon tetrachloride is also due to its metabolites formed in the hepatic SER. Experimental studies show that toxic changes in the SER can be detected within minutes of intravenous ingestion and are greatly enhanced by previous treatment with phenobarbital or with alcohol, a response that has long been recognized clinically (see section 7.2.6).

Drug-induced carcinogenesis may be reduced or enhanced by microsomal enzyme induction depending on whether the carcinogenic agent is the drug itself or a metabolite (Conney, 1971). For example, when 3'-methyl-4-dimethylaminoazobenzene is fed to rats, hepatomas readily develop, but this effect can be prevented by simultaneously giving polycyclic aromatic hydrocarbons. This would appear to be due to the fact that the latter agents induce the hepatic metabolism of aminoazo dyes. Similarly polycyclic hydrocarbons can diminish the carcinogenic properties of 9,10-dimethyl-1,2-benzanthracene while the microsomal enzyme inhibitor SKF 525-A can enhance its carcinogenesis. These observations have led to the challenging concept that it may be possible to reduce the frequency of malignancy in certain situations (for example, in smokers) by the administration of a non-toxic drug capable of inducing the metabolism of the offending carcinogen. However, the complexity of the problem is exemplified by the fact that some carcinogenic agents may be metabolized to both non-carcinogenic and carcinogenic metabolites, and that the respective enzyme pathways can be induced by the same inducing agent.

Certain drugs increase the frequency of unplanned pregnancies in women taking oral contraceptives. This is apparently due to enzyme induction leading to enhanced rates of hormone metabolism. Rifampicin administration increases four-fold the velocity of breakdown of ethinyl oestradiol (Bolt et al., 1974). Other agents that have been implicated include ampicillin and barbiturates (Mumford, 1974) and anticonvulsants (Janz and Schmidt, 1974).

4.4.10 Therapeutic Applications of Enzyme Induction

The rapid developments of recent years in our understanding of microsomal enzyme induction have contributed greatly to our understanding of some of the factors affecting drug dosage and toxicity (see sections 4.4.8, 4.4.9, 7.2). However, there have so far been disappointingly few new lines of therapy based on enzyme induction.

Phenobarbital has been shown to be of value in the treatment of infants with unconjugated hyperbilirubinaemia (Crigler and Gold, 1969). The half-life of bilirubin is decreased as a result of enhanced microsomal glucuronidation. The same rationale has been used in the administration of intravenous ethanol to expectant mothers in the last few days of pregnancy (Waltman et al., 1969). The effectiveness of barbiturates in lowering the serum concentration of bilirubin in some infants with congenital non-haemolytic jaundice suggests that such infants do not have a complete genetic block in their ability to synthesize the enzymes concerned in bilirubin conjugation. This is a stimulating observation, because it raises the possibility of treating some inherited disorders with an appropriate enzyme inducer. Many diseases are expressions of specific genetic disturbances affecting the synthesis or activity of enzymes that are important in normal metabolism. Examples of such hereditary enzymatic defects include galacto-saemia, glycogen storage disease, phenylketonuria and congenital non-haemo-lytic jaundice. The molecular abnormalities that form the bases for these inborn errors of metabolism are unknown but could include a faulty DNA, impaired translation of DNA to appropriate RNA, or a deranged translation of RNA on the ribosomes. If a defective DNA molecule were responsible, then presumably enzyme synthesis could not be induced. However, if the enzyme defect were due to an abnormal control of DNA expression or enzyme synthesis, then treatment with suitable inducing agents might be clinically useful. Possible examples of this are the enhanced metabolism of galactose in galactosaemic patients given proges-terone (Pesch et al., 1960) and the increased hepatic glucose-6-phosphatase activity in patients with glycogen storage disease given triamcinolone (Moses et al., 1966). However, in neither of these conditions was the drug found to be of significant therapeutic value.

More encouraging results have been obtained in a few patients with over-production of steroids. Werk et al. (1966) treated two patients with non-tumourous Cushing's syndrome and achieved biochemical and clinical improvement. Over three months, the plasma 17-hydroxycorticoids fell from 42 and $38\mu g/100ml$ to 12 and $15\mu g/100ml$ in these two patients. However, not surprisingly, the rate of cortisol secretion was not significantly affected. Similar therapeutic benefit has been obtained with the use of $o\rho'$-DDD in Cushing's syndrome (Bledsoe et al., 1964). The liver has other enzymes that are more specific for the metabolism of ketosteroids than the inducible microsomal hydroxylases. However, it is possible that these enzymes are easily saturated, so that increased levels of ketosteroids may then be handled by the mixed-function-oxidase system. By increasing the amount of these enzymes, the catabolism of steroid hormones could be increased.

The search for other therapeutic applications of enzyme induction have so far met with little success. The possible advantages and disadvantages of enzyme induction in carcinogenesis have been mentioned (see section 4.4.9). A number of drugs facilitate the removal of dieldrin from body fat stores. In liver disease, it might be hoped that 'liver function' could be improved by enzyme induction, but so far, inducing agents have not been shown to have any consistent therapeutic benefit in this situation.

4.5 Miscellaneous Factors

Innumerable factors will influence the activities of drug-metabolizing enzymes in any one situation. The influences of genetic factors (see section 4.3) and foreign compounds given intentionally or absorbed inadvertently from the environment (see section 4.4.1) have been discussed earlier. The availability of endogenous cosubstrates can be a limiting factor in some type II reactions. For example, high doses of salicylamide tend to deplete the available stores of sulphate. The conjugation of salicylamide then becomes dependent on the speed of formation of sulphate from cysteine (Levy, 1971). This in turn can be affected by the dietary protein intake. The biotransformation of other drugs competing for sulphate can then be secondarily impaired.

Laboratory studies have repeatedly provided examples of the variations in drug metabolism that can result from seemingly minor changes in protocol or in general laboratory methods. The importance of a clean environment was shown by one study in which hepatic drug metabolism in rats was reduced when urine and faeces were allowed to accumulate for one week instead of being removed twice daily (Vesell et al., 1973). The mechanism of this inhibition was unknown, although it was speculated that ammonia intoxication may have played a role. The environmental temperature can influence drug responses in a number of ways, including changes in drug absorption, tissue distribution, and drug metabolism (Fuhrman and Fuhrman, 1961). Exposure of male rats to a temperature of 4°C for 4 days decreased the sleeping time response to hexobarbital and meprobamate, apparently as a result of microsomal enzyme induction (Fuller et al., 1972).

Differences due to sex are well recognized (see Kato and Gillette, 1965). Male rats generally have a greater capacity for hepatic microsomal drug metabolism than female rats. The greater capacity of the former is reduced by castration and the low capacity of the latter is enhanced by testosterone so that androgen secretion is probably important. However, sex differences vary considerably with the diet and with the enzyme system being studied. Kato and Gillette (1965) found a 3-fold difference with aminopyrine and hexobarbital as substrates, but virtually no sex difference in the hydroxylation of aniline and zoxazolamine. Starvation of male rats impaired the activities of sex-dependent enzymes that metabolized aminopyrine and hexobarbital, but enhanced the activities of the sex-independent hydroxylation of aniline. By contrast, starvation of female rats increased the metabolism of all substrates. Thus the general tendency in acute starvation is a reduction in the differences due to sex. The sex differences are also impaired or enhanced by low protein and high protein feeding respectively (Kato, 1966).

Furner and Feller (1971) further investigated the effects of starvation on drug metabolism in different species (rats, mice and guinea pigs) and with different drugs. They found a stimulatory effect of starvation that varied with the drug studied within each species as well as different responses between species. Other factors influencing the rates of drug metabolism include age (Kato and Takanaka, 1968), strain (Furner et al., 1969), season (Seawright et al., 1972), hypothalamic function (Nair et al., 1970), time of day, degree of crowding, painful stimuli, and litter of origin (Vesell, 1968).

5. Ethanol Metabolism

5.1 Alcohol Dehydrogenase (ADH)

5.1.1 Introduction

The major pathway of ethanol metabolism involves the enzyme ADH (E.C. 1.1.1.1.) which is present in the hepatic cell sap (or cytosol). It catalyzes the formation of acetaldehyde coupled with the reduction of NAD:

$$CH_3CH_2OH + NAD^+ \longrightarrow CH_3CHO + NADH + H^+$$

The subsequent oxidation of acetaldehyde to acetate involves aldehyde dehydrogenase and is also coupled with the reduction of NAD. Since ethanol metabolism is almost obligatory, with no known major feedback control, a significant change in the hepatic NAD/NADH ratio occurs. As discussed subsequently, this change in redox potential affects those reactions which are also coupled to NAD/NADH and is largely responsible for many metabolic derangements produced by ethanol, including hepatic steatosis, lactacidaemia and hyperuricaemia.

Alcohol dehydrogenase was the first NAD-dependent enzyme to be purified from yeast (Negelein and Wulff, 1937). It was subsequently purified from horse liver by Bonnichsen and Wassen (1948). Partly because of its value as a model for NAD-dependent enzymes there is a huge volume of literature concerning ADH and the differences between the enzymes derived from human liver, from equine liver and from yeast (Sund and Theorell, 1963; Theorell, 1967; von Wartburg et al., 1963, 1964; Blair and Vallee, 1966; Mourad and Woronick, 1967; Lutstorf and Megnet, 1968).

5.1.2 Distribution

Alcohol dehydrogenases are widely distributed in nature. They have been reported to occur in many diverse animal species, including invertebrates and in a variety of plants and micro-organisms. The horse is the animal species with the highest known activity of ADH (Nyberg et al., 1953; Moser et al., 1969). The liver has long been known to be the organ with the highest activity of ADH (Leloir and Munoz, 1938). It accounts for 80—90 per cent of total human ADH with small amounts detectable in the gastro-intestinal tract and some other tissues (Bartlett and Barnet, 1949; Jacobson, 1952; Moser et al., 1969). Comparison of ADH activities in different tissues have to be interpreted with caution since, as discussed subsequently, the isoenzyme pattern of different organs varies as does the substrate specificity of the different isoenzymes. Thus with the use of ethanol alone as substrate, one could fail to detect ADH in various tissues. However, in a histochemical study involving 35 different alcohols as substrates, evidence for the presence of some slight ADH activity was found in almost all tissues (Ferguson, 1965; Ferguson et al., 1966).

5.1.3 Physicochemical Properties, Isoenzymes and Atypical Forms

The alcohol dehydrogenases of human, monkey and equine livers are zinc-containing metalloenzymes with a dimeric structure and molecular weights of approximately 80,000. They are basic proteins with a high content of lysine and arginine. ADH from horse liver contains four atoms of zinc per molecule of which two can be removed by dialysis or zinc-complexing agents with abolition of enzyme activity (Drum et al., 1967; Weiner, 1969). Human ADH contains only two zinc atoms, both of which appear to be essential for enzyme activity (Blair and Vallee, 1966).

The enzyme appears to comprise two similar polypeptide chains, each with a reactive -SH group in a cysteine residue (Harris, 1964). The dissociation of the dimer yields two subunits which are inactive but which can be recombined to form isoenzymes with slightly different characteristics (Pietruszko et al., 1969; Jornvall, 1970; Jornvall and Harris, 1970). The presence of different isoenzymes in both plants and animals is well documented (Grell et al., 1965; von Wartburg et al., 1965; Moser et al., 1968; Smith et al., 1971). In human livers, up to seven fractions of ADH can be determined by chromatography and electrophoresis. Furthermore in any one population, an atypical ADH can be distinguished from the normal ADH (von Wartburg and Papenberg, 1966; von Wartburg, 1971). However, the atypical ADH is subject to the same polymorphism as the normal enzyme and the atypical subfractions can be distinguished from the normal ones by their catalytic properties. Thus the pH optimum is 10.8 for the typical ADH and 8.5 for the atypical form and thiourea produces stimulation and inhibition respectively of the two enzymes. Such differences have been used to screen populations to determine the relative frequency of the different enzymes. The abnormal ADH was found in 20 per cent of a Swiss population and only 4 per cent of Londoners (von Wartburg, 1971). Some of the isoenzymes of the typical and atypical forms appear to be inter-convertible as a result of dissociation and recombination (Lutstorf and von Wartburg, 1969). It is conceivable that the kinetic properties of the atypical ADH are determined by the types of combinations of the subunits of the enzyme.

5.1.4 Substrate Specificity, Coupled Reactions

ADH has a remarkably broad substrate specificity (table VII). Its substrates include aliphatic, aromatic, cyclic, primary and secondary alcohols and their respective aldehydes and ketones (Theorell, 1965). A number of biogenic alcohols, such as those derived from serotonin and dopamine, are good substrates of ADH (von Wartburg, 1971). In view of the polymorphism discussed earlier, it is not surprising that there are differences in substrate specificity between species (as well as between individuals within the same species). Thus the demonstration that human ADH can oxidize methanol (von Wartburg et al., 1964) provided a rational basis for the observed value of ethanol in the treatment of methanol poisoning, a finding that was unexplained by the known substrate specificity of horse liver ADH. Single isoenzymes also show marked differences in their ability to oxidize the various substrates and there are similar differences between typical and atypical forms of human ADH (von Wartburg et al., 1965). Theorell et al. (1966) have isolated an ADH fraction with steroid-oxidizing ability; it catalyzes the oxidation-reduction of the primary alcohol group of sterols with a 3-β-hydroxy or a 3-keto group.

ADH can catalyze a number of other reactions. It has isomerase activity, accelerating the NAD-dependent conversion of glyceraldehyde phosphate to dihydroxyacetone phosphate (Van Eys, 1961). This activity may take place at a locus on the enzyme surface different from that for ethanol oxidation because inhibitors such as folic acid analogues (Vogel et al., 1964; Wada et al., 1967) and o-phenanthrolene and iodoacetate (Wallenfels and Sund, 1957) affect the two reactions differently. ADH can also catalyze the NAD-dependent interconversion

Table VII. Substrates of human liver alcohol dehydrogenase[1]

Substrate	Relative velocity
I. Alcohols	
Methanol	15
Ethanol	100
n-Propanol	103
Isopropanol	61
n-Butanol	113
Butanol, tertiary	0
Amyl alcohol	83
Isoamyl alcohol	79
Amyl alcohol, tertiary	30
1-Hexanol	80
3-Hexanol	48
n-Octanol	46
Ethylene glycol	8
1,2-Propandiol	76
Glycerol	25
Glycero-1-phosphate	0
Sorbitol	2
Cyclohexanol	67
Furfuryl alcohol	51
Benzyl alcohol	48
II. Aldehydes	
Formaldehyde	24
Acetaldehyde	100
Butyraldehyde	124
Isovaleraldehyde	100
Glyoxal	0
Pyruvate	0
Furfural	94
Cyclohexanon	6
Benzaldehyde	13
Anisaldehyde	4

1 Relative velocity = maximal activity with substrate/maximal activity with ethanol (or acetaldehyde), in percentage (from Wartburg, 1971)

of retinal and retinol (in the pathway of vitamin A metabolism). This reaction is normally ascribed to the enzyme retinene reductase, but the properties of the two enzymes are so similar that it is possible that they are the one enzyme (Koen and Shaw, 1966; Reynier, 1969; Koivusalo and Tarkkanen, 1969). ADH also takes part in coupled alcohol-aldehyde transhydrogenation reactions through its cofactor couple NAD/NADH (Redetzki, 1960):

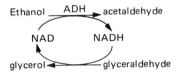

Similar reactions are involved in the enhanced activity of chloral hydrate (by accelerated conversion to trichloroethanol) and the hyperlactacidaemia (from conversion to pyruvate to lactate) that occurs during ethanol metabolism. Similarly ADH can facilitate other enzymes such as acetaldehyde dehydrogenase (AcDH) to produce a dismutation of an aldehyde with the formation of the corresponding acid and alcohol (Abeles and Lee, 1960; Lundquist et al., 1962a):

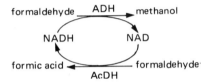

5.1.5 Regulation of the Rate of Ethanol Oxidation Via the ADH Pathway

Theoretically, a number of factors could affect the rate of ethanol oxidation in this pathway:

1) the amount of hepatic ADH
2) the type of hepatic ADH
3) competition with other substrates
4) rate of reoxidation of NADH.

A number of observations render the first two possibilities unlikely. Comparisons between species show no correlation between the measured quantities of hepatic ADH and the *in vitro* or *in vivo* rates of ethanol oxidation (Aebi and von Wartburg, 1960; von Wartburg and Eppenberger, 1961). Thus the rate of ethanol oxidation in the horse is much slower than in humans despite the considerably higher content of ADH in horse liver.

Similarly, the livers of subjects with the atypical enzyme have a total ADH activity four times greater than that of livers containing the typical enzyme, but there is no significant difference in the *in vivo* rates of ethanol metabolism (von Wartburg and Schurch, 1968; Edwards and Evans, 1967). Furthermore, the hepatic level of ADH is unaffected by some conditions that alter the rate of *in vivo* metabolism such as fasting (Smith and Newman, 1959) and the diurnal rhythm (Wilson et al., 1956).

The possibility that competing substrates affect the *in vivo* activity of ADH has received little attention. As discussed in the previous section, the substrate specificity of ADH is remarkably broad. Thus the equilibrium levels of a number of endogenous substrates could cause a stimulation or a competitive inhibition of the enzyme *in vivo* that would not be detected by an *in vitro* assay. For example, as discussed in section 6.5.2, a greater availability of glyceraldehyde (such as may follow heavy fructose ingestion) could conceivably enhance the rate of ethanol metabolism. Such a mechanism could conceivably be related to the observation that the rate of ethanol metabolism is greater in the fed than in the fasted state (Smith and Newman, 1959; Kinard et al., 1960). However, a more likely explanation would seem to be that depletion of glycogen in the fasted state impairs the generation of NADPH needed for the microsomal oxidation of ethanol (see section 5.3.5). This is consistent with the observations of Scholz et al. (1973) that mitochondrial inhibitors do not abolish the effects of fasting and feeding on rates of ethanol metabolism. Furthermore, corresponding changes are seen in the rate of metabolism of aminopyrine, a typical substrate for the NADPH-dependent microsomal drug detoxifying enzyme system.

The rate of reoxidation of NADH has received considerable attention as potentially the most important factor controlling the rate of ADH activity *in vivo* (Forsander, 1970; Hawkins and Kalant, 1972). The hepatic NAD/NADH ratio falls sharply and reproducibly during ethanol oxidation mainly as a result of an increase in NADH (Forsander et al., 1958; Smith and Newman, 1959; Cherrick and Leevy, 1965). Theoretically, reoxidation of NADH could be accomplished in three ways. First, there could be activation of cytosolic enzymes that are also coupled to the NAD/NADH ratio but which tend to move the ratio in the opposite direction to that produced by ADH. Such a mechanism probably accounts for the observed three- to four-fold increase in the rate of ethanol clearance (Lowe and Mosovich, 1965; Zuppinger et al., 1967) in patients with type I glycogen storage disease (glucose-6-phosphatase deficiency). The high hepatic pyruvate concentrations observed in such cases could enhance the reoxidation of NADH:

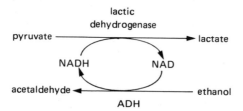

However, an alternative explanation for the enhanced rate of ethanol metabolism in this disorder is the increased hepatic content of glucose-6-phosphate. This could speed up the generation of NADPH, the cofactor of the microsomal ethanol oxidizing system.

A second mechanism for reoxidation of NADH could be transhydrogenation with NADP to form NADPH (Ernster and Lee, 1964). This could be of major importance in the regulation of the rate of ethanol metabolism because it could result in the maintenance of high concentrations of the cofactors for both the ADH and microsomal pathways.

The major mechanism for control of hepatic cytosolic NADH levels appears to be oxidation by the respiratory chain in the mitochondria. This could be limited by either the rate of transport of reducing equivalents into the mitochondria or by the rate of oxidation itself (which could be limited by lack of phosphate acceptor, or phosphate, for oxidative phosporylation). Changes in the respiratory chain are thought to occur in less than a second after the changes in the cytosolic redox state. This would indicate an extremely rapid transfer of reducing equivalents across the mitochondrial membrane, yet the latter is impermeable to NADH. To explain this paradox, a number of so-called shuttle mechanisms have been postulated (Krebs, 1967; Forsander, 1970). These involve the transfer of reducing equivalents across the mitochondrial membrane in the form of substrate pairs which are linked by a dehydrogenase which exists on both sides of the membrane. For example, one shuttle system can be depicted as follows:

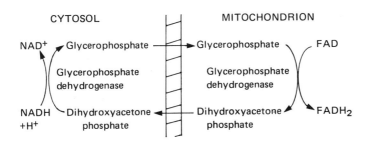

Both the glycerophosphate and the dihydroxyacetone phosphate cross the mitochondrial membrane barrier freely, and thus hydrogen equivalents can be rapidly delivered from reduced NAD directly to the flavoproteins of the electron transport chain, while the activity of glycerophosphate dehydrogenase ensures a rapid resupply of dihydroxyacetone phosphate for continuation of the cycle. Hepatic glycerophosphate has indeed been found to increase after ethanol administration (Nikkila and Ojala, 1963; Rawat, 1968) but Hassinen (1967)

reported little effect of this substrate pair on oxidation of NADH. Another shuttle mechanism is that of malate:

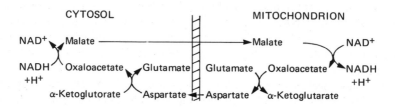

In this mechanism, hydrogen equivalents enter the mitchondrion via malate and are used to reduce intramitochondrial NAD which is then reoxidized by the electron transport chain. However, the mitochondrial membrane is impermeable to oxaloacetate so that a further conversion to ketoglutarate has to occur. This is catalyzed by the enzyme aspartate transaminase (or glutamic oxaloacetic transaminase or GOT) and is linked to yet another shuttle mechanism, namely that involving glutamate and aspartate (Chappell, 1968).

On the basis of these shuttle mechanisms it has been postulated that the *in vivo* rate of ethanol oxidation by ADH depends on the ability of the cell to maintain a normal NAD/NADH ratio and that this in turn is governed by the energy needs of the cell (supplied via the mitochondrial respiratory chain). In support of this view, Israel et al. (1970) and Videla and Israel (1970) found that 0.1mM dinitrophenol (which uncouples oxidative phosphorylation and enhances the rate of utilisation of hydrogen equivalents by the mitochondrion) increases the rate of ethanol oxidation in normal rat liver slices and *in vivo* by 100 to 160 per cent.

5.1.6 Biological Significance of ADH

In the drinking subject, ADH is the main pathway for ethanol clearance and the relative importance of this and of other enzyme systems is discussed in section 5.4. However, the biological significance of ADH in the non-drinking subject is unknown. One view (Theorell, 1965) is that the normal physiological role of this enzyme is the oxidation of one or more of its many naturally occurring substrates (see section 5.1.4). An alternative view (Wallgren and Barry, 1970; Krebs and Perkins, 1970) is that there are sufficient sources of endogenous ethanol especially in plant-eating mammals, to account for the preservation of the ADH system during biological evolution.

5.1.7 Endogenous Ethanol

Ethanol produced in the alimentary tract of humans and rats appears to result largely from bacterial activity and fermentation (McManus et al., 1966; Krebs and Perkins, 1970; Blomstrand, 1971). Ethanol can also be formed from glucose by some parasitic worms (Crompton and Ward, 1967). In addition, a number of steps in intermediary metabolism could theoretically result in aldehyde synthesis and subsequent conversion to ethanol by ADH (Krebs and Perkins, 1970). However, the blood levels of non-drinking humans and rats do not exceed 0.15mg per 100ml (Walker and Curry, 1966) and this ethanol could easily be eliminated via mechanisms other than ADH activity. However, in various other species, intoxicating blood levels of ethanol can be attained from alimentary fermentation of various plants (Krebs and Perkins, 1970). Thus ADH activity is by no means 'excessive' for the endogenous sources of ethanol in these species. It has been postulated that endogenous ethanol could produce malabsorption (see section 2.3.5) and could thus affect the response to ingested drugs.

5.2 Catalase

Catalase (E.C. 1.11.1.6) has long been known to be capable of catalyzing the peroxidative conversion of ethanol and other alcohols *in vitro* (Keilin and Hartree, 1945):

$$CH_3CH_2OH + H_2O_2 \longrightarrow CH_3CHO + 2H_2O$$

A H_2O_2-generating system is required. Rapid rates of ethanol and methanol oxidation can be achieved *in vitro*, but higher alcohols are poor substrates. Aminotriazole is an effective inhibitor. The enzyme is widely distributed in the body, especially in the liver, kidney and red cells. In the liver it is found mainly in the peroxisomes, which separate with the mitochondrial fraction of the cell on ultracentrifugation.

The significance of catalase in ethanol metabolism *in vivo* is unknown. The general consensus of opinion would appear to be that it plays no significant role. Most of the recent interest in catalase has followed the demonstration by Lieber and his associates of significant rates of ethanol oxidation in hepatic microsomes. There has been considerable controversy concerning whether this microsomal activity is due to a separate enzyme system or is due to microsomal contamination with catalase in the presence of some source of H_2O_2. As discussed in section 5.3.4, the controversy has been resolved by the demonstration (especially by chromatographic separation) of a distinct catalase-free microsomal enzyme system. However, this does not exclude the possibility that catalase may have some role to play in ethanol oxidation under certain circumstances. Trémolières and Carré (1960) described conditions in which the peroxidatic oxidation of ethanol could occur in the plasma *in vitro*. However, H_2O_2-generating systems sufficient to maintain such conditions are not known to occur either in health or in chronic alcoholism. Lundquist (1970) suggested that under pathological conditions, accelerated purine metabolism (for example via the xanthine oxidase system) might conceivably provide sufficient H_2O_2 to activate catalase:

$$\text{Hypoxanthine} + H_2O + O_2 \xrightarrow[\text{Xanthine oxidase}]{} \text{Xanthine} + H_2O_2$$

$$+$$

$$H_2O_2 + CH_3CH_2OH \xrightarrow[\text{Catalase}]{} CH_3CHO + 2H_2O$$

However, such a view is highly speculative and has no experimental basis. It is generally accepted that the H_2O_2 mediated peroxidation of ethanol by catalase is limited by the rate of H_2O_2 generated rather than by the amount of catalase. Many investigators have pointed out that the rate of peroxide formation in the liver is too low to involve catalase in appreciable ethanol oxidation. The physiological rate of H_2O_2 production is estimated to be 3.6μmole/hr/g of liver (Boveris et al., 1972). This could account for 2% of the *in vivo* rate of ethanol oxidation of 178μmole/hr/g of liver (Lieber and De Carli, 1972), assuming 3.5g of liver per 100g body weight. However, the above figure of 2% is probably an overestimate because not all of the hepatic H_2O_2 can be used by the peroxidatic reaction of catalase (Oshino et al., 1973). The microsomes account for almost half the hepatic generation of H_2O_2 (Boveris et al., 1972) yet this source of H_2O_2 does not contribute to ethanol oxidation in the perfused liver (Thurman and Scholz, 1973). Furthermore, the breakdown of the catalase-H_2O_2 intermediate by ethanol has a K_m of less than 0.6mM for ethanol (Theorell et al., 1972) which is more than one order of magnitude than the apparent K_m of the ADH-independent pathway of 8.8mM for ethanol *in vivo* (Lieber and De Carli, 1972).

5.3 Microsomal Ethanol Oxidizing System (MEOS)

5.3.1 Introduction

'The origin of an original work is always the pursuit of a fact which does not fit into accepted ideas'.
Claude Bernard, Manuscript, Collège de France.

The possible existence of the MEOS pathway was first suspected when electron microscopic studies showed a proliferation of the rat hepatic smooth endoplasmic reticulum after chronic ethanol feeding (Iseri et al., 1964). Such an increase in smooth endoplasmic reticulum resembles that seen after administration of a wide variety of xenobiotic compounds – including numerous drugs (Meldolesi, 1967; Conney, 1967) and food additives (Lane and Lieber, 1967). A feature common to most of these compounds is the fact that their metabolism takes place, at least in part, in the smooth endoplasmic reticulum itself. Until that time the only significant site of ethanol oxidation was thought to be in the hepatic cytosol as a result of ADH activity. These ultrastructural studies raised the possibility that ethanol might also be metabolized in the endoplasmic reticulum as well as in the cytosol. Subsequent studies have shown that a microsomal enzyme system capable of ethanol oxidation does in fact exist (Lieber and De Carli, 1968, 1970a). A number of properties distinguish it from ADH and from catalase (vide infra). It is characterised by being NADPH- and oxygen-dependent and sensitive to carbon monoxide:

$$CH_3CH_2OH + NADPH + H^+ + O_2 \longrightarrow CH_3CHO + NADP^+ + 2H_2O$$

Thus it has characteristics similar to those of many other hepatic microsomal drug-metabolizing enzymes.

5.3.2 Differentiation of MEOS from the Enzyme System Described by Orme-Johnson and Ziegler

Orme-Johnson and Ziegler (1965) reported that the microsomal mixed function oxidase system could catalyze the oxidation of methanol and ethanol to their corresponding aldehydes *in vitro*. However, the rate of ethanol metabolism by this system is very small, being only one-tenth that of MEOS (Lieber and De Carli, 1968, 1970a). The system described by Orme-Johnson and Ziegler oxidizes methanol at a rate twice that of ethanol, does not utilize higher alcohols and is insensitive to CO. By contrast, MEOS is twice as active for ethanol as for methanol, effectively oxidizes propanol and butanol, and is inhibited by CO (Lieber and De Carli, 1968, 1970a; Teschke et al., 1974b).

5.3.3 Differentiation of MEOS from ADH

Largely on the basis of studies with inhibitors, Isselbacher and Carter (1970) suggested that MEOS activity could be accounted for by microsomal contamination with cytosolic ADH during separation of the cell components. However, the specificities of the various inhibitors used are relative, so that variations in minor details of procedure can give very different results. A number of studies have since shown that MEOS is an enzyme system distinct from ADH.

1) Intracellular localisation. MEOS is microsomal whereas ADH is found in the cytosol (Lieber and De Carli, 1970a; Nyberg et al., 1953). Washed microsomes are capable of ethanol oxidation but have no detectable ADH activity, even when acetyl pyridine NAD (3-AP-NAD), which increases ADH activity (Kaplan et al., 1956), is added as a cofactor (Lieber et al., 1970).

2) Optimum pH. ADH has a pH optimum *in vitro* of 10 to 11 whereas that for MEOS is in the physiological range (Lieber and De Carli, 1968, 1970a).

3) Cofactor requirements. These also differ. ADH requires NAD, although *in vitro* some ADH activity with NADPH is possible (Dalziel and Dickinson, 1965). Using NADP or NADPH, alcohol oxidation cannot be detected in the cytosol despite its high ADH content (Isselbacher and Carter, 1970). Similarly, in the presence of NAD, little ethanol oxidation takes place in the microsomes (Lieber and De Carli, 1970a), and NADPH or a NADPH generating system is needed. Isselbacher and Carter (1970) claimed that NADPH could be replaced by 3-AP-NAD for microsomal ethanol oxidation but Lieber et al. (1970) could not confirm this.

4) O_2 requirements and CO inhibition. ADH and MEOS can also be differentiated by the latter's O_2 requirement and CO inhibition (Lieber and De Carli, 1968, 1970a).

5) Inhibitors. The well established role of pyrazole as an inhibitor of ADH has also been used to distinguish it from MEOS. Pyrazole is hepatotoxic in high concentrations and produces a number of ultrastructural changes with depression of cytosolic and microsomal enzyme activities (Lieber et al., 1970). Using a low concentration of pyrazole (1mM), Isselbacher and Carter (1970) reported a marked (48 per cent) decrease in MEOS activity. However, others (Lieber and De Carli, 1970a; Khanna and Kalant, 1970) found a relative lack of effect of low concentrations of pyrazole on MEOS and a striking inhibition of ADH. Thus 1mM pyrazole inhibited ADH activity *in vitro* by 98 per cent without significantly altering MEOS activity, and 2mM pyrazole produced inhibitions of 100 per cent and only 11 per cent respectively (Lieber and De Carli, 1970a).

6) Adaptive changes with chronic ethanol intake. These also distinguish MEOS from ADH. As discussed subsequently, MEOS, but not ADH, activity increased 2- to 3-fold after chronic feeding of ethanol (Lieber and De Carli, 1970a).

7) Column chromatography. This has also been used to confirm the differences between MEOS and ADH (see below). Teschke et al. (1974a) obtained from rat hepatic microsomes a MEOS-containing fraction. The absence of ADH in this fraction was confirmed by enzymatic assay and by complete insensitivity to 0.1mM pyrazole. Furthermore the apparent K_m of MEOS in this fraction was 7.2mM in contrast to the apparent K_m of ADH of 2mM. The addition of horse

liver alcohol dehydrogenase did not increase the rate of ethanol oxidation. A similar separation of ADH from MEOS activity was reported by Mezey et al. (1973).

5.3.4 Differentiation of MEOS from Catalase

There has been considerable controversy concerning whether the MEOS system is indeed a distinct and separate enzyme system or merely represents the activity of microsomal traces of catalase enhanced by the availability of H_2O_2 provided by NADPH oxidase. Much of the controversy has centred around the use of inhibitors to differentiate MEOS from catalase. A number of agents has been used to conclude that MEOS is indeed an enzyme system distinct from previously known pathways (Lieber and De Carli, 1968, 1970a, 1973a; Lieber et al., 1970). Thus cyanide 10^{-4}M inhibits MEOS by only 12–15 per cent but catalase activity is almost completely abolished (Lieber and De Carli, 1970a). Similarly 0.1mM azide *in vitro* or pyrazole 4.4mmoles per kg *in vivo* had little effect on MEOS but markedly inhibited microsomal catalase and microsomal ethanol oxidation by H_2O_2 derived from xanthine oxidase activity (Lieber and De Carli, 1970a; Lieber et al., 1970). Other studies have produced opposing or conflicting results (Isselbacher and Carter, 1970; Carter and Isselbacher, 1972; Khanna et al., 1970; Thurman et al., 1972; Lin et al., 1972). A major problem in interpretation of these studies is that none of the inhibitors are specific. Thus apparently minor alterations in protocol between various studies can lead to very different results. Cholate has been shown to reduce both NADPH oxidase activity and microsomal ethanol oxidation (Isselbacher and Carter, 1970) but cholate also inhibits a number of microsomal enzyme functions (Huttered et al., 1970). Aminotriazole (AT) has also been used to distinguish between the oxidation of ethanol by catalase and that by MEOS (Carter and Isselbacher, 1972). However, this agent has been shown by Kato (1967) and by Byron and Tephly (1969) to cause a general inhibition of microsomal drug metabolism with impairment of drug-induced stimulation of cytochrome P-450 synthesis.

In the former study, AT was given 5 times in the 24 hours before sacrifice, each time in a dose of 2g per kg. In the latter study, aminotriazole 3g per kg was given daily for 4 days. Carter and Isselbacher (1972) suggested that a single dose of aminotriazole 2g per kg one hour before sacrifice could be used to distinguish between the oxidation of ethanol by catalase and by MEOS, but data on the activity of NADPH oxidase under these experimental conditions were not provided. CCl_4 has been used *in vitro* to inhibit MEOS activity (Carter and Isselbacher, 1972). Only a small reduction in ethanol metabolism was achieved. However, the method used (conversion of ^{14}C-ethanol to ^{14}CO$_2$ by liver slices was unsuitable for assessment of ethanol metabolism because, as discussed in sections 5.6 and 9.5, very little ethanol is converted directly to CO_2 by the liver.

Even if inhibitors could reliably be shown to distinguish between NADPH-dependent MEOS and microsomal peroxidative mechanisms, it would not necessarily mean that the two systems are different. Hawkins and Kalant (1972) have speculated that the active site of the microsomal catalase could be more effectively protected by H_2O_2 from NADPH oxidase activity within the microsomes than by H_2O_2 generated in the soluble phase of the suspending medium.

With the chromatographic separation of MEOS from catalase (Teschke et al., 1972, 1974a) as well as from ADH (Teschke et al., 1972, 1974a; Mezey et al., 1973) the controversy and speculation concerning inhibitors has become less relevent. Using DEAE cellulose column chromatography and KCl gradients (fig. 6), a clear separation has been obtained of a fraction containing MEOS activity. This was free of catalic activity as assessed spectrophotometrically by failure of H_2O_2 to be consumed and by the absence of O_2 production in the presence of perborate (Teschke et al., 1972). There was also complete insensitivity of MEOS to 1.0mM azide and 0.1mM sodium cyanide, whereas both of these are potent inhibitors of the peroxidative activity of catalase (Teschke et al., 1974a). Furthermore, replacement of an NADPH-generating system with a H_2O_2-generating system failed to promote ethanol oxidation in the purified MEOS fraction, unless catalase was also added (table VIII).

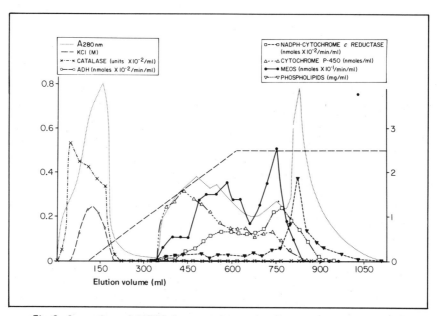

Fig. 6. Separation of MEOS from catalase and ADH activities by DEAE-cellulose column chromatography after solubilization of microsomes obtained from rats fed an ethanol containing liquid diet for 3 weeks. (From Teschke et al., 1972).

Table VIII. Effect of catalase and H_2O_2 generation on the ethanol oxidation catalyzed by a purified MEOS fraction (Teschke et al., 1974a)

Catalase (units)	Incubation system	Ethanol oxidation (nmoles acetaldehyde/ min/flask)
0	NADPH generated	16.4 ± 1.5
150	NADPH generated	24.4 ± 2.3
0	H_2O_2 generated	0
150	H_2O_2 generated	37.4 ± 2.9

Substrate specificity has also been used to distinguish MEOS from catalase. Orme-Johnson and Ziegler (1965) demonstrated microsomal oxidation of ethanol and methanol but not of alcohols with longer aliphatic chains. This was interpreted as evidence that catalase plays a role in microsomal ethanol oxidation (Thurman et al., 1972) because higher aliphatic alcohols are not substrates for catalase or at best, extremely poor ones. However, Teschke et al. (1974b) reported significant microsomal oxidation of propanol and butanol in the presence of NADPH, while at the same time confirming the low affinity of these alcohols for catalase-H_2O_2 (table IX). Chronic ethanol feeding in rats enhanced the microsomal oxidation of higher alcohols still further (table X). These studies, together with the results of column chromatography provide strong evidence for the catalase-independent nature of MEOS.

5.3.5 Microsomal Components of MEOS

Column chromatography has already contributed significantly to an understanding of MEOS, but preliminary investigations have not yet revealed the details of its composition. Teschke et al. (1974a) found MEOS activity only in purified fractions containing cytochrome P-450, NADPH-cytochrome *c* reductase and phospholipids. Activity could not be demonstrated in the absence of cytochrome P-450 but whether the presence of the other two components was essential could not be determined. Similar findings were obtained using microsomes from rats fed ethanol-containing diets for three weeks (Teschke et al., 1972). In that study, different peaks of MEOS activity could be obtained according to the concentration of the KCl used. These peaks may correspond to different forms of cytochrome P-450, with different specific activities (Joly et al., 1972; Comai and Gaylor, 1973). Form I of cytochrome P-450 is selectively induced by chronic ethanol intake (Joly et al., 1972; Comai and Gaylor, 1973) and has a much lower affinity for CO than form II. The latter is induced by phenobarbital (Comai and Gaylor, 1973). The inhibition of MEOS activity by CO (Teschke et al., 1974a) is somewhat lower than that of some other drug-metabolizing enzymes and this may reflect a role for form I of cytochrome P-450 in MEOS.

5.4 Chronic Ethanol Ingestion and Metabolic Tolerance to Ethanol

5.4.1 The Role of ADH

ADH activity following chronic alcohol consumption has been the subject of conflicting reports. There have been claims that hepatic ADH activity increased (Hawkins et al., 1966; Mistilis and Garske, 1969) or did not change, or even decreased (von Wartburg and Rothlisberger, 1961; Greenberger et al., 1965; Morrison and Brock, 1967; Videla and Israel, 1970; Lieber and De Carli, 1970a; Carulli et al., 1971; Singlevich and Barboriak, 1971; Raskin and Sokoloff, 1972). In some studies there was a moderate initial increase in ADH activity, but a subsequent return to normal or even a decrease with prolonged ethanol intake (Dajani et al., 1963; Figueroa and Klotz, 1962; Bode et al., 1970). Hepatic acetaldehyde dehydrogenase showed a similar but less marked response in one study (Dajani et al., 1963) but no change in others (Raskin and Sokoloff, 1972; Redmond and Cohen, 1971). Extrahepatic ADH, especially in the stomach, has been reported to be increased by alcohol (Mistilis and Garske, 1969), but others found no rise in gastric ADH after either acute or chronic ethanol feeding (de

Table IX. Substrate specificity of the microsomal alcohol oxidizing system. The incubations were carried out with systems generating either NADPH (0.4mM $NADP^+$, 8mM sodium isocitrate and 2mg per ml of isocitrate dehydrogenase) or H_2O_2 (10mM glucose and 0.7µg per ml of glucose oxidase). The values represent the average results of three experiments and are expressed as nmoles aldehyde/min/mg protein (Teschke et al., 1974b)

Substrate	NADPH	H_2O_2
Methanol	7.7	7.8
Ethanol	9.5	9.2
Propanol	4.6	0.2
Butanol	3.9	0

Table X. Effect of chronic ethanol consumption (6—8 weeks) on the activity of the microsomal alcohol oxidizing system. Female rats were pair-fed nutritionally adequate liquid diets containing either ethanol or dextrin as controls. The values represent means (± SEM) of six pairs (Teschke et al., 1974b)

Substrate	Control rat	Ethanol fed rat	p	Control rat	Ethanol fed rat	p
	nmoles aldehyde/min/ mg micros. protein			nmoles aldehyde/min/ 100g BW		
Methanol	7.3±0.6	12.7±1.0	<0.01	983±45	1650±83	<0.001
Ethanol	9.9±0.4	14.9±0.8	<0.01	1364±57	1948±83	<0.01
Propanol	5.8±0.6	11.1±0.9	<0.01	808±102	1461±150	<0.02
Butanol	4.4±0.3	7.4±0.7	<0.01	575±49	966±95	<0.01

Saint-Blanquat et al., 1972). Severe alcoholism in humans is associated with a general impairment of hepatic function due to the direct toxic effects of ethanol and/or to associated malnutrition. Under these conditions the activities of all pathways of hepatic ethanol metabolism could be impaired. In this regard, it is interesting to note that a low protein diet reduces rat hepatic ADH activity (Bode et al., 1970).

Actually the real question in assessing the role of ADH in the increased tolerance of alcoholics, is not what happens to ADH activity as assayed *in vitro,* but what happens to factors controlling the rate of reoxidation of NADH. The latter is regarded as the rate-limiting factor in ADH activity and, as discussed in section 5.1.5, there is little correlation between ethanol elimination *in vivo* and measurements of ADH activity. Theoretically, NADH oxidation could be accelerated in three ways:

1) There could be an increased concentration of substrates that require NADH for their metabolism in the cytosol (as has been postulated to be the case for the enhancement of ethanol metabolism by fructose). However, there is no evidence that such a mechanism could account for the increased rate of ethanol oxidation of alcoholics.

2) There could be an increased rate of transhydrogenation between NADH and NADPH, a mechanism that could link the ADH and microsomal ethanol oxidizing systems.

3) There could be an enhanced rate of NADH oxidation in the mitochondrial respiratory chain.

With regard to the third possible mechanism, a number of factors could accelerate the oxidation of NADH in the mitochondria. Uncouplers of oxidative phosphorylation such as dinitrophenol increase respiratory chain activity and have been shown to accelerate ethanol oxidation in liver slices (Videla and Israel, 1970). However, the relevance of this to *in vivo* ethanol metabolism remains to be elucidated. Hepatic oxidative phosphorylation after ethanol has been reported to be decreased (Banks et al., 1970), unchanged (Rubin et al., 1972), or variable (Pilstrom and Kiessling, 1972). Furthermore, the dinitrophenol effect did not persist in rats fed ethanol for 3–4 weeks and in which ethanol metabolism was increased by 70–90 per cent (Videla and Israel, 1970).

Activity of the mitochondrial respiratory chain could also be increased by an improved transfer of hydrogen equivalents from NADH across the mitochondrial membrane. The latter is normally impermeable to NADH. As discussed elsewhere (French, 1971; Hawkins and Kalant, 1972; Lieber, 1973a) ethanol produces numerous structural and functional changes in the hepatic mitochondria of humans and animals. In one study, mitochondrial permeability to NADH was reported to be increased by ethanol (Rawat and Kuriyama, 1972). However, the rates of NADH oxidation were very high in the control mice of their study, suggesting that the experimental conditions had produced mitochondrial damage. Ethanol feeding makes the mitochondria more susceptible to *in vitro* damage during cell fractionation (Rubin et al., 1970). Thus the differences reported in NADH oxidation rates in the above study may have been artefactual. Furthermore, there was no increased mitochondrial permeability after ethanol feeding in another study in which isoosmotic conditions were maintained (Cederbaum et al., 1972). Another way in which the transfer of hydrogen equivalents from cytosolic NADH into the mitochondria could be accelerated would be by an enhancement of 'shuttle' systems across the mitochondria (see section 5.1.5). There is no evidence that ethanol does in fact affect these shuttle systems. However, this mechanism may be the explanation for the enhanced rate of ethanol metabolism in rats given the hypocholesteraemic agent, clofibrate (Atromid-S). There is an associated 5-fold increase in activity of α-glycerophosphate dehydrogenase which could represent stimulation of the corresponding shuttle system (Kahonen et al., 1971).

5.4.2 The Role of Catalase

Catalase activity in humans is not increased by chronic ethanol intake (Ugarte et al., 1972). In rats, some groups found no change (von Wartburg and Rothlisberger, 1961; Hawkins et al., 1966; Lieber and De Carli, 1970a), but Carter and Isselbacher (1971a) reported an increase. However, as in the case of ADH, the pertinent question is whether chronic ethanol feeding affects the rate limiting factor in enzyme activity. For catalase, this appears to be the rate of H_2O_2 generation rather than the amount of available catalase (Portwich and Aebi, 1960). However, the chronic intake of ethanol enhances the activity of

NADPH-oxidase (Lieber and De Carli, 1970b; Carter and Isselbacher, 1971a). Thus the latter enzyme could increase the availability of H_2O_2 for peroxidative metabolism by catalase:

$$
\begin{array}{l}
\rule{0pt}{1em}\text{NADPH} + \text{H}^+ + \text{O}_2 \xrightarrow{\hspace{2cm}} \text{NADPH}^+ + \text{H}_2\text{O}_2 \\
\hspace{3.5cm}\text{NADPH} \\
+ \hspace{3.4cm}\text{Oxidase} \\
\\
\text{H}_2\text{O}_2 + \text{CH}_3\text{CH}_2\text{OH} \xrightarrow{\hspace{2cm}} 2\text{H}_2\text{O} + \text{CH}_3\text{CHO} \\
\hspace{3.5cm}\text{Catalase}
\end{array}
$$

However, the studies of Thurman and Scholz (1973) indicate that this pathway plays no part in ethanol oxidation *in vivo*. Furthermore, as discussed in section 5.2, catalase generally appears to be of negligible importance in ethanol metabolism *in vivo*.

5.4.3 The Role of MEOS

The role of MEOS in the enhanced ethanol tolerance of alcoholics is also controversial. However, the bulk of the evidence indicates that MEOS plays a significant part. This view is based on the observed SER proliferation associated with chronic ethanol intake and on direct and indirect evidence of enhanced MEOS activity.

1) SER proliferation. Iseri et al. (1964) first observed that alcohol intake produces a striking proliferation of the smooth endoplastic reticulum. This has been confirmed by further studies in rats (Iseri et al., 1966; Rubin et al., 1968) in primates (Pieper et al., 1972; Lieber et al., 1973; Rubin and Lieber, 1974) and in humans (Lane and Lieber, 1967; Rubin and Lieber, 1967; Lieber and Rubin, 1968; Rubin and Lieber, 1968a). By contrast, Dobbins et al. (1972) applied morphometric analysis to electron micrographs of rat livers and concluded that ethanol feeding decreased the surface area of the smooth endoplasmic reticulum. However, this conclusion was based on the counting of intersections of membranes with superimposed grid lines, a method that fails to take into account the effect of possible changes in shape of the endoplasmic reticulum. Furthermore, biochemical estimation of microsomal phospholipid and protein have confirmed that ethanol feeding does result in an increased mass of smooth endoplasmic reticulum (Ishii et al., 1973).

2) Direct evidence of enhanced MEOS activity. MEOS activity is also increased by chronic ethanol feeding and Lieber and De Carli (1972) have calculated that, when corrected for microsomal losses during the preparative procedure, the rise in MEOS activity could account for one-half to two-thirds of the observed increase in blood ethanol clearance. Lieber (1973a) has suggested that

the remainder of the rise in ethanol clearance may be due to enhanced ADH activity. This could be related to changes in MEOS activity in two ways. First, there might be accelerated reoxidation of NADH for the ADH pathway as a result of greater availability of NADPH from MEOS activity since the NADP/NADPH systems are linked (Veech et al., 1969). Second, NADH could serve as a partial donor of electrons for microsomal drug-detoxifying pathways (Cohen and Estabrook, 1971b). In this regard it is interesting to note that the addition of ethanol to hepatic microsomes produced a modified type II binding spectrum, the magnitude of which is tripled by ethanol feeding (Rubin et al., 1971). The hepatic MEOS activity of mice did not fall on withdrawal of ethanol in one study (Rawat and Kuriyama, 1972), but the method used for assay of MEOS is questionable and has not been validated. A more satisfactory method of MEOS assay has been used to show that activity of this enzyme is increased by ethanol feeding (Reed and Mezey, 1972) and does return to normal after ethanol withdrawal (Mezey and Tobon, 1971). There was a rough correlation between MEOS activity and blood ethanol clearance if changes in liver size are taken into account; by contrast, there was an inverse relationship between ethanol clearance and hepatic ADH activity (Mezey and Tobon, 1971; Shah et al., 1972).

3) Indirect evidence. Indirect evidence for a significant role of MEOS in the enhanced ethanol tolerance of alcoholics is supplied by consideration of other aspects of hepatic microsomal metabolism. For example, observed changes in hepatic lipoprotein production and in total body energy requirements after chronic ethanol intake (see sections 6.2.3, 6.10) can be linked to enhanced microsomal oxidation of ethanol. Similarly, other drugs (such as barbiturates) which increase MEOS activity (Lieber and De Carli, 1970c) also accelerate blood ethanol clearance (Fischer, 1962; Lieber and De Carli, 1972; Mezey and Robles, 1974). These findings were not confirmed in a number of other studies (Tephly et al., 1969; Klassen, 1969; Roach et al., 1972; Khanna et al., 1972). However, the apparent conflict can be largely explained by consideration of the experimental conditions. Thus, in some studies, long-acting barbiturates were used and ethanol clearance was tested soon after the last dose of barbiturate. Under these circumstances, blood barbiturate levels were probably raised, and competition for binding to cytochrome P-450 could interfere with ethanol metabolism (Lieber and De Carli, 1972). In some experiments, ethanol was given intraperitoneally for the clearance studies. This route of administration is unsatisfactory for such studies because it causes chemical peritonitis and necrosis of the liver, especially at its surface (Strubelt et al., 1972). In one study (Khanna et al., 1972) ethanol clearance did increase by 11.5 per cent after phenobarbital treatment but this did not attain statistical significance. The drugs whose administration enhanced MEOS activity in rats were phenobarbital, butylated hydroxytoluene and 3-methylcholanthrene (Lieber and De Carli, 1970c). However the increase was only evident when enzyme activity was expressed per 100g body

weight. MEOS activity per mg of microsomal protein was not increased in contrast to the significant rise that followed ethanol feeding. These findings are in keeping with a study of Mezey and Robles (1974) in four alcoholic patients. Phenobarbital significantly increased the clearance of ethanol but the activity of MEOS (expressed per mg of total hepatic protein) was not increased. However, it is difficult to interpret negative findings in such a small series. It should be noted that ethanol and phenobarbital raise the levels of different forms of cytochrome P-450 (see section 3.4.4) and this *in vitro* finding would be expected to have some corresponding differences *in vivo*.

5.5 Acetaldehyde Metabolism

5.5.1 Aldehyde Dehydrogenase

The second step in ethanol metabolism, the disposal of acetaldehyde, occurs rapidly within the liver; it is not rate limiting and only slight rises in the levels of acetaldehyde in the blood are detectable (Wallgren and Barry, 1970; Truitt and Walsh, 1971). A very large number of enzymes is capable of metabolizing acetaldehyde but the main pathway involves oxidation to acetate (von Wartburg, 1971), mainly under the action of aldehyde dehydrogenase (E.C. 1.2.1.3). The latter is located principally in the mitochondria, with some activity present in cytosol and in microsomes (Grunnet, 1973). In the liver, two aldehyde dehydrogenases with similar properties can be separated chromatographically from the cytosol (Kraemer and Deitrich, 1968; Shum and Blair, 1971). Because these enzymes are NAD-dependent, their activity further contributes to the disturbed NAD/NADH ratio produced by the ADH activity.

5.5.2 Oxidases

Oxidases such as xanthine oxidase (E.C. 1.2.3.1) and aldehyde oxidase (E.C. 1.2.3.2) are also capable of oxidising acetaldehyde with production of H_2O_2 (Rajagopalan and Handler, 1964). Theoretically the H_2O_2 produced could be used by catalase for the oxidation of ethanol. However, the results of *in vitro* studies suggest that this pathway of acetaldehyde metabolism is of little significance under physiological conditions.

5.5.3 Lyases

A number of lyases are known to be capable of catalyzing condensation reactions between acetaldehyde and other compounds, thus providing a mechanism for acetaldehyde disposal without oxidation. Little is known of these reactions and they are thought to be of little significance in the metabolism of ethanol. The reactions are reversible and provide potential sources of acetaldehyde for the endogenous production of ethanol by ADH. Acetoin is formed from condensation of pyruvate with acetaldehyde (Stotz et al., 1944). The level of acetoin in the serum is increased in hepatic coma (Soling et al., 1964) but is not appreciably affected by ethanol metabolism (Hassinen, 1963). Other lyases acting on acetaldehyde result in condensation with α-ketoglutarate to form 5-hydroxyhexanoic acid (Bloom and Westerfeld, 1966) with glyceraldehyde-3-phosphate to form 2-deoxyribose-5-phosphate (Racker, 1952), and with glycine to form threonine (Karasek and Greenberg, 1957).

5.6 Metabolism of the Acetate Formed from Ethanol

Acetate is the major product of ethanol oxidation and further metabolism takes place predominantly in other tissues. This was first suggested by Lundsgaard (1938) and Leloir and Munoz (1938) and subsequently confirmed by a series of elegant Scandinavian studies. Forsander et al. (1960) showed that the isolated rat liver oxidizes ^{14}C-ethanol efficiently but incompletely with only 2–7 per cent recovered as CO_2 whereas a perfused hind-limb preparation oxidizes very little ethanol, but does so completely. However, when the hind-limb was perfused with a medium that had been through the liver, the production of $^{14}CO_2$ was much increased. In human subjects with hepatic venous catheters, Lundquist et al. (1962b) showed that most of a dose of administered ethanol leaves the liver as acetate. Similar conclusions were reached from studies with isolated perfused animal livers and hepatic slices (Forsander and Räihä, 1960; Lundquist et al., 1963; Gordon, 1968). The impaired capacity of the liver to utilize acetate results from the inhibition of hepatic Krebs cycle activity (see section 6.2.1).

Once it has left the liver, the acetate derived from ethanol appears to be used as effectively as that derived from other sources (Lieber and Davidson, 1962; Smith, 1961). Within 2 hours of the clearance of ethanol from the blood, 85 per cent of it has been eliminated to CO_2 (Bartlett and Barnet, 1949; Burbridge and Hine, 1951; Schiller et al., 1959). Some is lost directly in urine and expired air, and much of the remainder is incorporated into the tissues. Watanabe et al. (1966) reported that 3–6 per cent of a single injection of labelled ethanol was incorporated into the tissues of mice.

5.7 Racial Differences in Ethanol Metabolism

Genetic factors could influence the responses to a dose of ethanol in two main ways. One would be by altering the blood concentration achieved (because of inherited differences in absorption or metabolism). The other would be by altering the response to the same blood concentration of alcohol. Interest in this subject stems partly from the observed social differences in the acute responses to drinking and in the incidence of alcoholism. An example of the former is the facial flushing that may be associated with drinking alcohol. It is a commonly held view that this is more common amongst Orientals than amongst people of European origin. This view was tested by Wolff (1972). Beer drinking visibly affected only one out of 34 adult Caucasians but produced marked facial flushing in 65 of 82 adult Japanese, Taiwanese and Koreans. This was confirmed by a more objective measurement, namely optical densitometry of the earlobe, which showed significant increases in 64 of the Orientals but in only two of the Caucasians. Similar differences in vasomotor responses were also found in infants tested with a solution of port wine in glucose. The Oriental adults also had a significantly higher incidence of subjective symptoms such as palpitations, tachycardia and dizziness after alcohol. Unfortunately the study appears to have been poorly controlled with regard to degree of fasting and dosage of alcohol. Most Caucasians received more beer per gm body weight than the Orientals. Furthermore, blood levels of alcohol were not recorded, so it is not known whether the greater susceptibility to the effects of alcohol of one group was due to a slower clearance of ethanol or to a difference in response to the same blood concentrations. The fact that the vasomotor changes appeared within a few minutes and reached a peak in half an hour of drinking suggests that blood alcohol levels were not critical.

There is no experimental evidence for an inherited difference in responses to a known blood alcohol level but the list of possibilities is endless. Racial differences in autonomic responses to drugs are known to occur (La Du, 1969; Vesell, 1969) and similar variations might apply to ethanol. Ethanol might conceivably stress an enzyme system that is congenitally deficient and turn a compensated state into a clinical syndrome. Such a situation would be analogous to the effects of drugs such as quinidine in producing haemolytic anaemia in persons with G6PD deficiency. Alternatively, ethanol might 'normalize' an inherited metabolic defect. For example, compared to controls, alcoholics have a lower urinary excretion of tryptamine (Schenker et al., 1966) and higher urinary levels of VMA (Kissin et al., 1973). Both these abnormalities tend to return to normal with ethanol ingestion. This is of interest because it suggests a 'normalizing' influence of ethanol on the metabolism of biogenic amines, compounds that have been implicated in the development of alcoholism. As pointed out by Kissin (1974a), apart from such biochemical differences, there is a whole range of parameters — physiological, neurophysiological, behavioural and psychological — in which alcoholics differ from non-alcoholics. However, whether these differences are due to hereditary influences or to environmental factors (such as prolonged alcohol intake) remains a matter of conjecture.

Genetically determined differences in the rate of ethanol metabolism could theoretically affect the response to drinking. Sporadic examples of this are seen in patients with type I glycogen storage disease (see section 5.1.5), but very little has been written about possible ethnic variations in the rate of ethanol metabolism. This was the subject of an intriguing Canadian study comparing Canadian whites with Eskimoes and Indians (Fenna et al., 1971). The investigation was prompted by sporadic medical and law-enforcement reports that Indians jailed while drunk took longer to become sober than whites in similar conditions. To exclude the possible effects of congeners and of different rates of absorption, ethanol was given intravenously. The subjects were Eskimoes, Indians and Canadian whites with normal liver function tests. The native Canadians were found to have a significantly slower clearance of ethanol. The 50 per cent difference could not be correlated with previous drinking or dietary habits and the authors concluded that genetic factors were probably responsible. A puzzling feature of this study was the finding that alcohol clearance in whites did not differ significantly between those classed as heavy drinkers and those classed as light. This contrasts with the metabolic adaptation to drinking shown by the native Canadians, with a 50 per cent higher ethanol clearance in heavy drinkers than in light ones. It is also at variance with the findings of the New York study of Misra et al. (1971) that whites studied under metabolic ward conditions showed a significant increase in ethanol clearance after a period of controlled alcohol intake. This raises the question of whether the two groups in the Canadian study may have differed in regard to other environmental factors, such as exposure to drugs and other chemicals that could stimulate microsomal ethanol oxidation. The Eskimoes and Indians were mainly patients convalescing from fractures or infections, whereas the whites were mainly staff members. A repetition of this study under metabolic ward conditions might help to elucidate this question.

Metabolic differences in responses to alcohol are of special interest because of their potential relevance to the development of alcoholism. In Australia, alcoholism is a much greater problem amongst aborigines than amongst the other population groups (who themselves are not noted for their abstention). In the United States, American Indians are specially prone to alcoholism in contrast to the low incidence amongst Jews. Such ethnic variations are generally ascribed to cultural, social and economic factors. Inherited differences in the activity of hepatic alcohol dehydrogenase *in vitro* are well known but these are not accompanied by corresponding changes in ethanol elimination. Nevertheless, the possibility remains that genetically determined factors could influence the metabolic responses to ethanol and a considerable amount of energy has been expended in the studies of animals inbred for their preference for alcohol. As pointed out by Lieber (1972a), the findings of Fenna et al. (1971) suggest that groups with a high incidence of alcoholism, such as American Indians, have a low rate of ethanol metabolism; thus attempts to correlate ethanol preference in animals with an enhanced rate of ethanol metabolism may not be relevant to the problem of alcoholism in humans. It may be that the capacity for metabolic adaptation (by microsomal enzyme induction) may be more important.

5.8 Extrahepatic Metabolism of Ethanol

The liver is undoubtedly the major site of ethanol oxidation. Its central role in a variety of species has been shown by studies in eviscerated and hepatec-tomized animals, in perfused livers, and in tissue slices and homogenates (Wallgren and Barry, 1970), and in human studies using ^{14}C-ethanol (Bartlett and Barnet, 1949). Larsen (1959) calculated that approximately half the elimi-nation of ethanol in human subjects could take place outside the liver. However, his studies were all carried out at blood concentrations of alcohol below 5mg per 100ml, a condition of little relevance to the average drinker. Carter and Issel-bacher (1971b) reported that rat gastro-intestinal slices oxidize ethanol at a rate one-fifth to two-thirds that of hepatic slices studied under the same conditions. However, the method used in this study gave extremely low results for both tissues, presumably because only the total conversion of ethanol to CO_2 was estimated (see section 9.5). The small amount of extrahepatic metabolism of ethanol that does occur is thought to be in part due to ADH in other tissues. ADH activity is found in the kidney (Leloir and Munoz, 1938; Bartlett and Barnet, 1949; Jacobson, 1952), gastro-intestinal tract (Spencer et al., 1964) and seminal vesicles (Ferguson, 1965), and to a lesser extent in most other tissues. As discussed in sections 5.1.6 and 5.4.1, the biological significance of ADH is uncer-tain and its role in heavy drinking is unknown. Reports that gastro-intestinal ADH activity is enhanced by chronic ethanol intake have not been confirmed. MEOS has been demonstrated in adipose tissue (Scheig, 1971) and it would be of interest to know if its activity there can be enhanced by ethanol in the same manner as occurs in the liver.

5.9 Miscellaneous Pathways of Ethanol Metabolism

The biotransformation of ethanol by minor pathways has been shown to occur, but its quantitative significance is not known. From in vitro studies of maximum rates of ethanol metabolism, it would seem that extremely little ethanol is handled by these other routes. Fatty acid ester formation has been demonstrated in vitro (Newsome and Rattray, 1965) and in vivo (Goodman and Deykin, 1963). Small amounts of ethanol can also be excreted in the urine as sulphates and glucuronides (Hawkins and Kalant, 1972). As discussed by these latter authors, competition with other drugs for conjugating pathways could theoretically result. However, there is no evidence that this does in fact occur.

6. General Metabolic and Pharmacological Consequences of Ethanol Metabolism

6.1 Relationship to Other Factors in Alcoholism

Before discussing some of the complications of ethanol metabolism, it is worth considering the role played by other factors in the clinical problems associated with drinking alcohol. Because of the diversity of such factors, alcoholism can be associated with an extraordinary variety of clinical manifestations. For example malnutrition may account for the development of some specific syndromes (particularly in the nervous system). These are often due to poor dietary intake, but secondary gastro-intestinal disturbances (possibly aggravated by direct effects of ethanol) may produce varying degrees and types of malabsorption and contribute further to the disturbed nutritional state. The congeners of alcoholic beverages may be important, although more often than not their incrimination is based on conjecture. (An exception was the outbreak of 'alcoholic cardiomyopathy' in Quebec which was traced to the introduction of large amounts of cobalt into the beer from a local brewery). It is generally thought that genetic factors may also greatly influence the mode of presentation of the alcoholic. This view is reinforced by the observation that some people appear to be especially susceptible to one or other of the complications of alcoholism, while other individuals seem to be able to drink large amounts with impunity. However, as in the case of the congeners, the role of hereditary influences is largely based on speculation and is poorly documented. Finally, the social and economic problems of the alcoholic greatly influence the development of complications. For example, a high incidence of trauma and hypothermia (due to exposure) may predispose to the development of pancreatitis, while an enhanced susceptibility to drug addiction may affect hepatic function because of the attendant hazards of viral hepatitis, septicaemia and drug interactions.

Because of the difficulties in studying such factors under controlled conditions, it is not surprising that research into the complications of ethanol metabolism (involving relatively precise biochemical and physiological methods) has far outstripped research into other aspects of alcoholism. Naturally, this applies especially to the liver which bears the brunt of the metabolic disturbances produced by ethanol. This research activity has led to a shift in clinical emphasis. Some twenty to thirty years ago, it was fashionable to regard malnutrition as the major factor in alcoholic liver disease. Largely as a result of the work of Lieber and his associates, direct toxic effects of ethanol on the liver have been established (Rubin and Lieber, 1968a), and there has been a corresponding tendency to downgrade the importance of the diet. In this regard, it is important to bear in mind that there is simply no direct evidence that alcoholic liver disease is due, even in part, to malnutrition. However, it would be unfortunate if the excellent studies of Lieber's group were taken out of context and resulted in an excessive swing towards neglect of nutritional factors. The demonstration that ethanol, even with an adequate nutritional intake, can produce hepatic disease in humans (and in different animal models), does not exclude the possibility that malnutrition plays some part in alcoholic liver disease. It is well established that alcoholics are frequently malnourished and that malnutrition can in some circumstances be associated with hepatic disease. Furthermore, other complications of alcoholism, such as Wernicke's encephalopathy, are due to dietary disturbances. Thus until further information is available, it seems reasonable that the maintenance of an adequate or even an enriched diet should remain an important part of the treatment of the alcoholic.

6.2 Lipid Metabolism

The disturbances of lipid metabolism produced by ethanol have been the subject of a vast outpouring of papers in the past fifteen years. In the following sections, these will be reviewed very briefly under the headings of four major mechanisms. These are the changes in redox potential, mitochondrial damage, alterations in microsomal function and the roles of the diet and the intestine. The bulk of the views put forward is based on experimental work carried out by Lieber and his associates and details of references to these experiments may be found in reviews by Lieber (1973a, 1974).

6.2.1 Changes in Redox Potential

The major pathway of ethanol metabolism involves the enzyme ADH in the cytosol. The reduction of the associated cofactor, NAD, results in a prompt and marked change in the NAD/NADH ratio. This is aggravated by the subsequent conversion of acetaldehyde to acetate. The NAD/NADH ratio is of considerable importance to the cell because it governs the direction of a number of reversible oxidation-reduction reactions. It may at first seem surprising that a change in redox (reduction-oxidation) potential should occur so readily. No other commonly taken drug produces such changes. However, unlike most other pathways involving the NAD/NADH couple, there is no known feedback control for ADH. Also, unlike other sources of calories, ethanol cannot be stored. Furthermore, ADH has a low K_m (2mM or 9mg per 100ml). Thus, it is fully saturated following quite modest intakes of alcohol. Finally, no other drug is taken in such vast quantities as ethanol.

Thus for some hours after a moderate drinking episode, there are important changes in intermediary metabolism within the hepatic parenchymal cells (fig. 7). First of all, the increased supply of NADH in the cytosol is almost

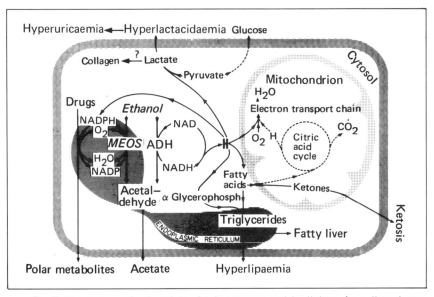

Fig. 7. Metabolism of ethanol in the hepatocyte and its link to fatty liver, hyperlipaemia, hyperuricaemia, hyperlactacidaemia and ketosis (ADH = alcohol dehydrogenase, MEOS = microsomal ethanol oxidizing system). Pathways that are decreased by ethanol are represented by dashed lines. (From Lieber, 1973b).

immediately reflected by a corresponding change within the mitochondria. The mitochondrial membrane is impermeable to NADH and the change appears to result from various 'shuttle' mechanisms (see section 5.1.5). At the same time, citric acid cycle activity is depressed, partly because some of its reactions are inhibited by the change in redox potential. In the fasting state, citric acid cycle activity is mainly dependent on a supply of two-carbon fragments derived from fatty acids. This normally supplies the NADH for the mitochondrial respiratory chain which in turn is the major source of ATP production for the cell. Thus in the presence of alcohol, the main fuel supply of the cell is diverted from fatty acid oxidation to ethanol oxidation.

The enhanced NADH/NAD ratio that inhibits fatty acid oxidation also favours triglyceride accumulation. This can arise in two ways. First, the conversion of dihydroxyacetone phosphate to α-glycerophosphate is favoured and the latter combines with fatty acids to form triglycerides. However, in contrast to the effects of a single dose of ethanol, its chronic consumption does not raise the hepatic α-glycerophosphate level. More importantly, fatty acid synthesis is enhanced, possibly by transhydrogenation to NADP or possibly by the mitochondrial elongation pathway. Thus there is an increased supply of both the fatty acid and glycerol components of the triglyceride molecule.

6.2.2 Mitochondrial Damage

Mitochondrial changes, in addition to those due to an altered redox potential, appear to be important in the disturbed lipid metabolism of the alcoholic. Morphological abnormalities of the hepatic mitochondria in alcoholics are well documented and include swelling and disfiguration, disorientation of the cristae and intra-mitochondrial crystalline inclusions. These ultrastructural changes are associated with enhanced mitochondrial permeability and fragility and decreased phospholipid content. The disturbances are due, at least in part, to ethanol itself, as shown by a number of carefully controlled studies in rats, baboons and human volunteers, including alcoholics and non-alcoholics. They also occur in association with high protein, low fat and choline-supplemented diets. The mechanism of these changes is unknown. It may be related to a depression of mitochondrial protein synthesis by ethanol. The change in redox potential that is produced acutely by ethanol is also present during chronic feeding, but rapidly returns to normal when ethanol is withdrawn (Gordon, 1972). However, the ultrastructural changes persist. These more prolonged morphological changes may play some part in the enhanced ketogenesis of the alcoholic which is most marked in the absence of ethanol. The mitochondrial changes may also contribute directly (independently of the altered redox potential) to the inhibition of fatty acid oxidation. Mitochondria from ethanol-fed rats were incubated *in vitro* in the absence of ethanol and were found to have a reduced capacity to oxidize fatty acid. However, β-oxidation was enhanced and this possibly accounts for the accelerated ketogenesis.

6.2.3 Alterations in Microsomal Function

Microsomal changes due to ethanol probably also contribute to the disturbed lipid metabolism of the alcoholic. The endoplasmic reticulum is the site of fatty acid esterification and lipoprotein production. Chronic ethanol intake enhances the activity of hepatic microsomal L-α-glycerophosphate acyl transferase, a key enzyme in triglyceride synthesis. The production of the protein moiety of lipoproteins is also increased, as is the activity of glycosyl-transferase, an enzyme of the Golgi apparatus involved in lipoprotein production. Chronic ethanol feeding also increases lipoprotein production even when ethanol is not present at the time of testing. This latter observation suggests that there is an enhanced capacity for lipoprotein production possibly related to the proliferation of the endoplasmic reticulum that is associated with microsomal ethanol oxidation. In addition, the acute effects of ethanol on fatty acid synthesis and oxidation (see earlier) could also favour lipoprotein production. The severity of the hyperlipaemia seen in the alcoholic is quite variable. This possibly reflects, in part, the variations in dietary lipid, and in the duration and dosage of ethanol as well as the presence of associated hepatic disease. Occasionally a very exaggerated response to alcohol is seen and this may be due to a forme fruste of some associated condition such as essential hyperlipaemia, diabetes, pancreatitis or an increased susceptibility to ethanol itself. Chronic ethanol intake increases the hepatic level of cholesterol ester, especially when taken with a cholesterol-free diet (Lefèvre et al., 1972). The mechanism may be related to increased microsomal enzyme activity as appears to be the case for the barbiturates. In addition, when ethanol is taken with cholesterol-containing diets, cholesterol catabolism is reduced and bile acid turnover is decreased (Lefèvre et al., 1972).

6.2.4 The Role of Diet and the Intestine

The role of dietary factors in the disturbed lipid metabolism has been the subject of vigorous debate. Part of the controversy has concerned the relative importance of dietary fatty acids and fatty acid mobilisation from adipose tissue in the development of the alcoholic fatty liver. It has now been shown that a single large dose of ethanol can both stimulate fatty acid mobilisation (by enhanced catecholamine release) or depress it (as a result of acetate produced in the liver from ethanol). The net effect may depend on the experimental conditions, and differences in this may account for some of the conflicting reports.

In any event, studies involving a massive single dose of ethanol are of little relevance to the effects of chronic alcohol consumption. In the latter circumstances, the fatty acids that accumulate in the liver appear to be mainly of dietary origin.

Another point of controversy has been the role of protein and lipotropic factors (methionine and choline) in the pathogenesis of the alcoholic fatty liver. Unfortunately, much of the early experimental work on this subject was done in the rat which shows significant species differences from humans in regard to choline metabolism. In humans, fatty livers are readily produced by ethanol alone, in the absence of protein deficiency and even in the presence of massive choline supplementation of the diet. These findings do not exclude the possibility that protein deficiency may aggravate the changes produced by ethanol. By contrast, the effects of changes in dietary fat are well established. The severity of alcoholic fatty liver is favoured by increasing the amount of dietary fat and by including long chain, rather than medium chain, fatty acids in the diet. Another area of interest has been the part played by intestinal lipoprotein production in alcoholic hyperlipaemia. A single large dose of ethanol has been shown to enhance the intestinal production of lipoprotein. However, subsequent studies revealed that the intestine appears to play no role in the hyperlipaemia due to chronic alcohol intake (except for a 'permissive' role in supplying dietary sources of lipid for utilisation by the liver).

6.3 Hyperlactacidaemia, Hyperuricaemia and Acidosis

Alcoholic excess is a well-known precipitating factor in gouty arthritis. Alcoholics readily develop a hyperuricaemia which is distinguishable from the primary variety by its reversibility when drinking is stopped. The sequence of events responsible for this predisposition to gout is as follows (Lieber et al., 1962). The raised NADH/NAD ratio increases the lactase pyruvate ratio in the hepatic parenchymal cell and results in a raised serum lactate because of the combined effects of decreased utilisation and hepatic production. Hyperlactacidaemia lowers the urinary excretion of uric acid and this results in hyperuricaemia. The increased blood lactate level also affects the plasma pH and contributes to the acidosis resulting from the increased ketogenesis.

6.4 Collagen Accumulation and Cirrhosis

That alcoholism leads to cirrhosis is common knowledge, but the mechanism of this association has defied investigation. This has been partly due to the failure to achieve, until recently, an animal model that mimics this disease of humans (Rubin and Lieber, 1974). It is commonly speculated that fatty liver, though readily reversible, represents a severe metabolic disturbance (as indicated for example by the mitochondrial changes). In its more severe form, this may be manifested by actual cell death and a secondary inflammatory reaction (alcoholic hepatitis). This in turn might promote scarring and fibrosis leading to cirrhosis. This hypothetical sequence of events remains unproven.

Cirrhosis and collagen accumulation are not synonymous. Nevertheless, the latter is a major feature of cirrhosis and there is considerable interest in the mechanisms promoting it. The hepatic collagen content is raised by prolonged ethanol consumption in rats and baboons. Hepatic collagen is in a dynamic state so an increase could result from enhanced synthesis, decreased breakdown, or both. Little is known about the control of collagen degradation. One could hypothesise that it is reduced by ethanol as a result of impaired lysosomal hyaluronidase activity or as a result of the appearance of hyaluronidase-resistant glycosaminoglycans (Huttered and Bacchin, 1968). With regard to an enhanced collagen synthesis, the raised NADH/NAD ratio could contribute by promoting hyperlactacidaemia; this in turn stimulates the activity of peptidyl-proline hydroxylase. An increased activity of this enzyme is a regular accompaniment of raised collagen synthesis. Prolonged feeding of ethanol to rats and baboons enhances hepatic peptidyl-proline hydroxylase activity as well as the incorporation of proline into hepatic collagen (Feinman and Lieber, 1972). Another finding of interest is the rise in the hepatic levels of new collagen and of glycosaminoglycuronans in patients with alcoholic hepatitis and cirrhosis (Galambos and Shapira, 1973). These findings are suggestive of the presence of fibroblastic activity, yet the cirrhotic livers showed minimal histological evidence of parenchymal necrosis and inflammatory exudate. These authors postulated that cell damage might initiate fibroblastic activity in alcoholic hepatitis and that some unknown mechanism might cause this to continue even after the ethanol was withdrawn (possibly as a result of altered mononuclear cell activity).

6.5 Carbohydrate Metabolism

The disturbances in glucose metabolism produced by alcohol are discussed in section 7.3.2 together with the interactions between ethanol and hypoglycaemic agents.

6.5.1 Effects of Ethanol on Fructose and Sorbitol Metabolism

The rate of fructose metabolism by the isolated perfused liver is not altered by ethanol (Damgaard et al., 1973), but the pattern of its utilisation is significantly changed (fig. 8). The production of glucose, lactate and D-glyceraldehyde is reduced and the outputs of glycerol and sorbitol increase to reach a new steady state. The formation of sorbitol is favoured by the altered NAD/NADH ratio due to ADH activity and in addition, fructose-1-phosphate accumulates suggesting an inhibition of aldolase activity (Damgaard et al., 1973).

Sorbitol metabolism is impaired by ethanol (Hillbom and Lindros, 1971). This has been shown by a reduced blood clearance of sorbitol in man (Verron, 1965) and by impaired oxidation of sorbitol in animals and in liver slices in the presence of ethanol (Hillbom, 1968). The mechanism of these effects is presumed to be the change in NAD/NADH ratio secondary to ADH activity.

6.5.2 Effects of Fructose on Ethanol Metabolism

The effects of fructose on ethanol metabolism are much better documented. Fructose has been shown to increase the rate of ethanol metabolism in human subjects and in various laboratory animals in a number of *in vitro* and *in vivo* models (Carpenter and Lee, 1937; Hawkins and Kalant, 1973; Damgaard et al., 1973). The magnitude of the effect varies with the species and some workers were unable to demonstrate it in the isolated perfused rat liver (Papenberg et al., 1970; Ylikahri et al., 1971). Holzer and Schneider (1955) suggested that glyceraldehyde formed from fructose could serve as a substrate for aldehyde dehydrogenase and enhance the rate of reoxidation of NADH (fig. 8). Theoretically, during ethanol and fructose oxidation, glyceraldehyde metabolism might be diverted from glycerate to glycerol as a result of the raised cytosolic NADH/NAD ratio and as a result of competitive inhibition of glyceraldehyde oxidation by acetaldehyde. The latter is to be expected because the K_m of aldehyde dehydrogenase for acetaldehyde (Deitrich et al., 1962) is much less than that for glyceraldehyde (Sestoft et al., 1972). This view is supported by observations of the enhanced rate of hepatic ethanol oxidation when glyceraldehyde is added to pig liver perfusates (Damgaard et al., 1973) and by the enhanced rate of glycerol production when liver slices were incubated with fructose and ethanol (Thieden and Lundquist, 1967; Rawat, 1970).

However, Damgaard et al. (1973) dispute this view on the grounds that under steady state conditions no net formation of glycerol (or of sorbitol) takes place. These reduced metabolites only accumulate during the transient stage when fructose levels are increasing. Furthermore, they were unable to detect an increased concentration of metabolites of glycerol such as 1-glycerol 3-phosphate or triglycerides, although one wonders if their experimental conditions were suitable for the detection of an increase. These authors provided evidence for an alternative hypothesis, namely, that NADH is reoxidised by transhydrogenation to form NADPH. The latter could then be used in other metabolic

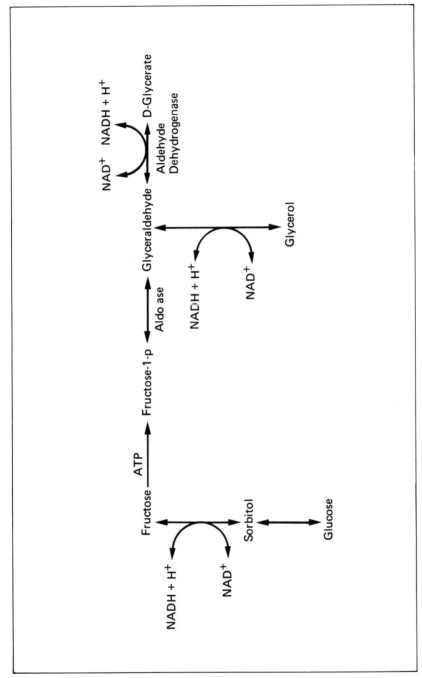

Fig. 8. Scheme of some of the main steps in fructose metabolism.

pathways such as in microsomal ethanol oxidation and in the conversion of acetate (from ethanol) to fatty acids.

6.5.3 Effects of Ethanol on Galactose Metabolism

Galactose tolerance has been used as a standard test of hepatic function in the past. Ethanol markedly impairs the removal of galactose from the circulation and increases its urinary excretion. The mechanism of this effect is an inhibition of the hepatic enzyme uridine diphosphate-galactose epimerase secondary to the increase in the NADH/NAD ratio produced by ADH activity (Isselbacher and Krane, 1961). Thus the inhibition is dependent on the actual presence of ethanol but is independent of the blood level of ethanol above concentrations of 10mg per 100ml (Tygstrup and Lundquist, 1962). A comparable inhibition is produced by the metabolism of sorbitol which, like that of ethanol, also raises the NADH/NAD ratio.

6.6 Miscellaneous Metabolic Disturbances

A number of other metabolic disturbances are associated with alcohol intake. A discussion of these is beyond the scope of this book and the reader may wish to refer to other more detailed publications (Wallgren and Barry, 1970; Kissin and Begleiter, 1971, 1974). *Protein metabolism* is frequently disturbed in the alcoholic as a result of hepatic parenchymal dysfunction and malnutrition. In addition, ethanol directly inhibits hepatic protein synthesis (Jeejeebhoy et al., 1972). The mechanism of this effect is unknown. It may be related to the reduction in hepatic RER produced by ethanol (Ishii et al., 1973). The *renal* effects of ethanol are also poorly understood. Despite the presence of ADH in the kidney, the chronic consumption of ethanol does not alter the renal levels or ratio of NADH and NAD (Kalant et al., 1970). Thus renal ADH activity has no known role in the renal accumulation of triglyceride produced by chronic ethanol intake (Lieber et al., 1966). In the *heart,* fatty change, and a number of other structural and functional changes can be produced by ethanol but their mechanism is obscure and a direct link to the metabolism of ethanol has not been established. A number of *haemopoietic* disturbances are seen in alcoholism. Numerous mechanisms are involved, including nutritional factors and direct toxic effects of ethanol but, as in the case of the myocardial changes, a relationship to ethanol metabolism has not been established. Changes in *serotonin* metabolism are common in alcoholism. The mechanisms are complex. Nutritional factors and direct effects of ethanol are involved. Urinary 5-hydroxy indole acetic acid is reduced and 5-hydroxytryptophol formation is enhanced.

This may result from ethanol oxidation and the associated changes in the NADH/NAD ratio and the raised acetaldehyde concentration. Catecholamine secretion is stimulated by large doses of ethanol, either as a nonspecific response to stress or as a result of raised concentrations of acetaldehyde. An enhanced NADH/NAD ratio in the cell favours the reductive pathway of norepinephrine metabolism, leading to an increased urinary level of glycol; there is a corresponding shift from the oxidative pathway, leading to a reduced level of 3-methoxy-4-hydroxyphenylglycolic acid (VMA).

6.7 Inhibition of Microsomal Drug Metabolism by Ethanol and Other Drugs

Persons under the influence of alcohol are more susceptible to the actions of a variety of drugs. This is most obvious in the case of sedatives and is thought to be largely due to an additive or synergistic effect in the central nervous system. However, studies of the effects of combined ethanol and amylobarbitone administration in the rat indicated that an increased drug susceptibility could precede central nervous system potentiation (Ratcliffe, 1969). This increased drug susceptibility could be partly due to the observed inhibitory effects of ethanol on the metabolism of a variety of drugs in vitro (Rubin and Lieber, 1968b; Rubin et al., 1970a; Rubin et al., 1970b; Ariyoshi et al., 1970; Mallov and Baesl, 1972).Corresponding to these in vitro studies, the simultaneous administration of ethanol with other drugs results in a decreased rate of metabolism of the drugs in vivo (Fischer, 1962; Rubin et al., 1970b; Carulli et al., 1971; Mallov and Baesl, 1972). Conversely, in the presence of drugs, ethanol metabolism is impaired (Whittlesey, 1954; Lieber and De Carli, 1972).

Our understanding of the possible mechanisms for the inhibition of drug metabolism by ethanol is incomplete. The experimental designs of the above studies exclude the possibility of non-specific hepatic dysfunction associated with alcoholic liver injury, but clearly this could play an additional role in some clinical situations. In the case of microsomal aniline hydroxylase, the inhibition is of a competitive nature (Rubin et al., 1970b). It may be related to the binding of ethanol to microsomes which has been shown to yield a modified type II spectrum (Rubin et al., 1971). This binding could result in interference with the microsomal binding of other drugs. Furthermore, like type II binders, ethanol inhibits the reduction of cytochrome P-450 (Rubin et al., 1970b) and this in turn could slow the entire chain of microsomal electron transport involved in drug metabolism. The mechanism of the inhibition of ethanol metabolism by other drugs is unknown. It seems reasonable to expect that there could be competition at a microsomal level, but such a view at present is only speculative. As in the case of chlorpromazine (see section 7.3.1), the ADH pathway could be involved in some instances.

6.8 Stimulation of Microsomal Drug Metabolism by Ethanol and Other Drugs

In contrast to their greater susceptibility when intoxicated, sober alcoholics have an increased tolerance to other drugs (Soehring and Schuppel, 1966; Carulli et al., 1971). This has generally been attributed to an increased tolerance of the central nervous system secondary to repeated alcohol intake (Forney and Hughes, 1968; Kalant et al., 1970; Hatfield et al., 1972). However, the dissociation that is sometimes observed between altered drug sensitivity and altered central nervous system tolerance (Ratcliffe, 1969) raises the possibility that there may also be a change in the rate of the metabolism of drugs. Indeed, alcoholics admitted to hospital and tested in the absence of ethanol have an accelerated rate of clearance of ethanol and other drugs (Kater et al., 1969b; Kater et al., 1969a). Conversely, asthmatic patients have an increased clearance of blood ethanol, an observation that may be due to the chronic intake of drugs by these patients (Sotaniemi et al., 1972). Of course, the changes in drug metabolism in the alcoholic can be due to a large number of factors other than ethanol itself. These include malnutrition, congeners of alcohol and an associated high intake of other drugs. However the intake of ethanol alone with a nutritionally adequate diet under metabolic ward conditions resulted in a striking increase in the blood clearance of meprobamate and of pentobarbital (Misra et al., 1971). This was demonstrated in both alcoholic (fig. 9) and non-alcoholic subjects and similar findings were obtained in rats. Similarly, ethanol intake has been shown to accelerate the metabolism of aminopyrine (Vesell et al., 1971) and of tolbutamide (Carulli et al., 1971).

These *in vivo* observations are clearly due, at least in part, to an accelerated hepatic microsomal metabolism of drugs and not just due to changes in distribution or excretion. Drug-induced hypertrophy of the smooth endoplasmic reticulum is a well recognized phenomenon that is usually associated with an increase in microsomal protein and enhanced activities of microsomal drug-metabolizing enzymes (Conney, 1967). As discussed earlier, ethanol ingestion also results in a proliferation of the smooth endoplasmic reticulum. Thus it is not surprising that a functional counterpart to this proliferation exists and that chronic ethanol intake in man and rats increases the activity of a variety of microsomal drug-metabolizing enzymes (Rubin et al., 1968b; Rubin et al., 1970a; Ariyoshi et al., 1970; Misra et al., 1971; Carulli et al., 1971; Mallov and Baesl, 1972; Joly et al., 1973). Thus hepatic slices and hepatic microsomes from rats fed ethanol for four weeks had an increased capacity to metabolize meprobamate (Misra et al., 1971) and CCl_4 (Hasumura et al., 1974).

The microsomal contents of phospholipid, cytochrome P-450 and NADPH – cytochrome P-450 reductase are also increased by ethanol feeding (Ishii et al., 1973; Joly et al., 1973). These compounds are known to play a key role in the

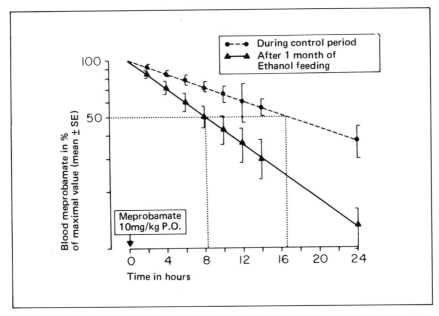

Fig. 9. Effect of ethanol consumption on blood clearance of meprobamate. Four alcoholic volunteers were tested before and after one month of ethanol ingestion. Half-lives are shown by the dotted lines on the x and y axes. (From Misra et al., 1971).

microsomal metabolism of a number of drugs (Lu et al., 1972). It is possible that they play a similar role in microsomal ethanol oxidation and its enhancement by chronic ethanol feeding. Teschke et al. (1972) chromatographically separated a microsomal fraction containing MEOS activity. In this there was an apparent correlation between the activities of MEOS and of NADPH-cytochrome *c* reductase, when phospholipids and sufficient amounts of cytochrome P-450 were present (fig. 6). However, other mechanisms could be responsible for the ethanol oxidation of this system. For example, cytochrome P-450 has significant peroxidative properties (Hrycay and O'Brien, 1971) and thus cytochrome P-450 (or a similar compound) might oxidize ethanol by this mechanism. Hassinen and Ylikahri (1972) reported that cytochrome P-450 in isolated perfused livers was reduced by aminopyrine but not by ethanol (when tested under the same conditions). This is in keeping with the observation that ethanol inhibits the reduction of cytochrome P-450 (Rubin et al., 1970b) in contrast to type I substrates such as aminopyrine which promote its reduction. Thus the finding is not unexpected and cannot be used to argue against a microsomal role for ethanol metabolism. However, it does not exclude the possibility that cytochrome P-450 may be involved. In any event, the increased activities of microsomal drug-detoxifying enzymes and the greater content of microsomal P-450 that follow chronic ethanol intake provide a rational explanation for the observed enhancement of drug metabolism *in vivo*.

6.9 The SER and Ethanol Dependence

A possible link between ethanol dependence and microsomal ethanol oxidation has been postulated by Lieber (1972b). The possible sequence of events (fig. 10) is as follows:

1) Chronic ethanol consumption stimulates the activity of MEOS and of the microsomal drug-metabolizing enzymes and leads to a proliferation of the SER.

2) The capacity for the metabolism of endogenous substrates is thus

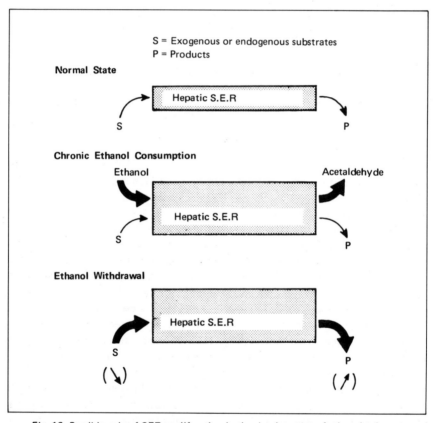

Fig. 10. Possible role of SER proliferation in the development of ethanol tolerance and dependence and in the interaction of ethanol with drug metabolism. (From Lieber, 1972b).

increased, but an actual increase in their biotransformation does not occur because of the presence of the competing exogenous substrate (ethanol).

3) On withdrawal of alcohol, the metabolism of the endogenous substrates is accelerated and produces untoward effects.

4) These effects can be alleviated by further drinking, thus promoting a craving for alcohol.

The postulated endogenous substrate (or substrates) responsible are not known and the hypothesis is not put forward as the sole mechanism for addiction. The principal determinants of dependence probably reside in the nervous system. Obviously, a number of neuroendocrine, psychological, socio-economic, and possibly genetic, factors are involved. However, the proposed theory is consistent with a number of observed changes associated with dependence. It also raises the possibility of new therapeutic approaches to the difficult problem of drug dependence.

6.10 Changes in Energy Requirements Associated with the Metabolism of Drugs, Including Ethanol

'La réspiration est donc une combustion' — *Lavoisier*

Microsomal drug metabolism is metabolically inefficient. The basis for this is that in microsomal drug oxidations, there are two substrates, the drug itself and NADPH, each losing some of their chemical energy and utilizing O_2 directly without the formation of a high energy compound such as ATP.

$$RH + NADPH + H^+ + O_2 \longrightarrow ROH + NADP^+ + H_2O$$

Presumably the chemical energy lost is dissipated as heat and, if not required for the body's thermoregulation, represents waste of energy. This metabolic inefficiency contrasts with the situation that applies in the case of the oxidation of most physiological substrates through the respiratory activity of the mitochondrial electron transport chain. This can be shown in abbreviated form as follows:

In the respiratory chain, a series of steps are interposed between the oxidation of the substrate and the utilization of O_2 with production of water. These steps are linked to synthesis of the high energy compound ATP so that instead of chemical energy being explosively lost as thermal energy, a high proportion is retained for its orderly use by the organism. In the case of glucose, approximately 42% of the free energy resulting from its combustion is captured in the form of high-energy phosphate and much of the remainder is lost as heat. Of course, whether the administration of a drug can cause a degree of metabolic inefficiency that is quantitatively significant for the whole organism will depend on a number of factors. These include (1) the enzyme pathways involved in clearance of the drug, (2) its caloric value and the caloric value of endogenous substrates whose oxidation by microsomal pathways might be enhanced by the administration of the drug, and (3) whether it is capable of inducing hepatic microsomal enzymes.

6.10.1 Ethanol Calories Do Not (Fully) Count

When ethanol is burned in a bomb calorimeter, it is found to have a caloric value of 7.1kcal/g. At the turn of the century, Atwater and Benedict (1896) carried out a series of classical physiological experiments which indicated that the calories of ethanol are used by the body as efficiently as those of carbohydrate or fat. Numerous studies have since served to strengthen this traditional view (Le Breton, 1936; Barnes et al., 1965; Wallgren and Barry, 1970). However, sporadic observations have been at variance with this concept (Mitchell and Curzon, 1940; Trémolières and Carré, 1961; Permon, 1962a; Saville and Lieber, 1965; Pirola and Lieber, 1972). In one report, the records were analyzed of 12 subjects studied under metabolic ward conditions who received ethanol (up to 50% of ingested calories) as an isocaloric substitution for carbohydrate (Pirola and Lieber, 1972). Their body weights showed a slight but steady fall, the mean daily weight change differing significantly from that during a stable pre-alcohol observation period (fig. 11). One might anticipate that this effect of ethanol might be enhanced if the intake of ethanol could be increased by giving ethanol as an addition to the diet rather than as an isocaloric substitution. This was indeed found to be the case in two further subjects studied (Pirola and Lieber, 1972). In one of these subjects, an increased dietary intake, supplying an extra 2,000 kcals per day resulted in the predicted increase in body weight (fig. 12). By contrast when the same number of additional calories were supplied as ethanol, there was no sustained rise in body weight (fig. 13). Other authors have studied the effects of ethanol on metabolic rates but the results have been conflicting. The possible explanation for these apparent contradictions is discussed below.

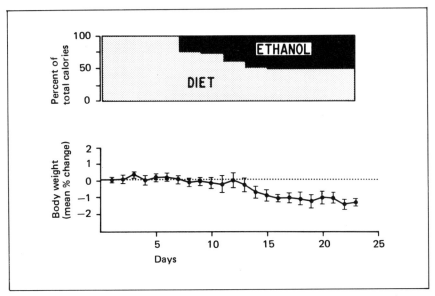

Fig. 11. Body weight changes after isocaloric substitution of carbohydrate (50% of total calories) by ethanol in 11 subjects (means ± standard errors). The dotted line represents the mean change in weight in the control period. (From Pirola and Lieber, 1972).

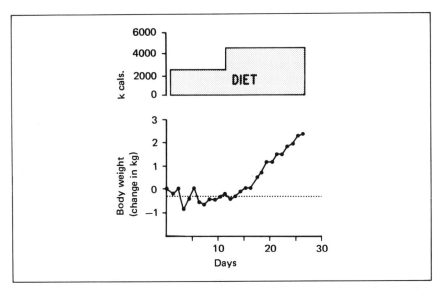

Fig. 12. Effect on body weight of adding 2,000 kcal/day as chocolate to the diet of the same subject as in figure 13. The dotted line represents the mean change during the control period. (From Pirola and Lieber, 1972).

6.10.2 Mechanism of Wastage of Ethanol Calories: Inefficient Microsomal Metabolism

'I had rather heat my liver with drinking'
William Shakespeare — Antony and Cleopatra.

One possible explanation for the wastage of ethanol calories referred to above could be that inefficient pathways of microsomal metabolism are involved, particularly after the chronic ingestion of high doses of ethanol (Pirola and Lieber, 1972). A comparison of the MEOS and ADH pathways demonstrates the differences in energy conservation (referred to earlier) between microsomal and mitochondrial oxidations.

$$CH_3CH_2OH + NADPH + H^+ + O_2 \xrightarrow[\text{MEOS}]{} CH_3CHO + NADP^+ + 2H_2O$$

$$CH_3CH_2OH + NAD^+ \xrightarrow[\text{ADH}]{} CH_3CHO + NADH + H^+$$

The oxidation of ethanol by the ADH pathway is efficient and comparable to that of, for example, lipids. For every mole of ethanol oxidized, a mole of NADH is produced and the oxidation of this in the mitochondrial election

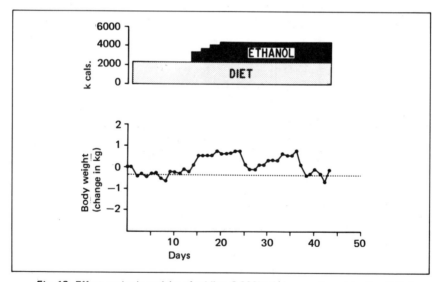

Fig. 13. Effect on body weight of adding 2,000kcal/day as ethanol to the diet of one subject. The dotted line represents the mean change during the control period. (From Pirola and Lieber, 1972).

transport chain produces 3 moles of ATP. By contrast, in the MEOS pathway, both ethanol and NADPH are oxidized without any apparent energy-conserving mechanism. In assessing the quantitative significance of this for the whole organism, a number of factors have to be taken into account:

1) The caloric intake in the form of ethanol can be huge; intakes of 500 kcal per day are common and ethanol calories may represent 50 per cent of the total caloric intake of the alcoholic.

2) The liver is thought to account for 20–25 per cent of the body's oxygen requirements.

3) Ethanol metabolism occurs mainly in the liver and has no known mechanism of feedback control.

4) During the oxidation of ethanol, the latter replaces fatty acids as the main metabolic fuel of the liver.

5) The quantitative significance of MEOS in ethanol metabolism is debatable, but it has been estimated that up to 50 per cent could be accounted for in this pathway, the exact amount depending on the blood concentration and on prior intake.

6) Other microsomal enzyme activities are induced by ethanol, such as the oxidation of NADPH (Lieber and De Carli, 1970b):

$$NADPH + H^+ + O_2 \xrightarrow{\hspace{2cm}} NADP^+ + H_2O_2$$
$$\text{NADPH}$$
$$\text{Oxidase}$$

6.10.3 Comparisons with Other Studies

The concept that the body's energy requirements are increased by ethanol is supported by the findings of Trémolières and Carré (1961). They reported that alcoholics had a 23 per cent higher basal metabolic rate than did controls. Furthermore, intravenous ethanol produced a rise in O_2 consumption above basal levels of 7 per cent in normal subjects and of 45 per cent in alcoholics without cirrhosis (in whom increased MEOS activity would be expected). More-over, a rise of only 8 per cent after ethanol was observed in alcoholics with cirrhosis (in whom some dysfunction of the endoplasmic reticulum might be expected). The apparent contradiction between these findings and those of some other authors (table XI) may be due to differences in the dose of ethanol and in the previous exposure to alcohol. As discussed earlier, the K_ms for ADH and MEOS are 2 and 8.6mM respectively corresponding to blood levels of 9 and 40mg/100ml. Thus a high dose of ethanol given to alcoholics with microsomal enzyme induction would be expected to produce the greatest rise in oxygen consumption. Similarly a low dose of ethanol such as that used by Atwater and Benedict (table XI) would not be expected to result in blood levels sufficient to saturate MEOS. Furthermore, because their subjects were not alcoholics,

Table XI. Effect of ethanol on oxygen consumption in human studies. Authors are listed in order of descending dose of administered ethanol

Investigators	Subjects	Route of adminis- tration	Ethanol dose g/kg	Oxygen con- sumption % change after ethanol
Learoyd, 1972[a]	alcoholic	oral	1.0	+20
Trémolières and Carré, 1961	normal	oral	0.7	+9
	alcoholic	oral	0.7	+28
	normal	intravenous	0.4	+7
	alcoholic	intravenous	0.4	+45
Barnes et al., 1965[a]	d	oral	0.4	+1.8
Perman, 1962[a]	normal	oral	0.3	+7.9
Carpenter and Lee, 1937[a]	normal	oral	0.22	+3.5
Winkler et al., 1963	d	intravenous	b	+10.4
Atwater and Benedict, 1896	normal	oral	0.17	0[c]

a   These studies were not carried out under basal conditions.
b   Ethanol was infused at a rate of 2.5mmoles/min which for a 70kg man would be equivalent to 0.1g/kg in 1h. Fructose was given with the ethanol and this would be expected to increase the rate of ethanol metabolism. Controls received fructose alone.
c   Numerous studies were carried out in 3 volunteers under varied conditions. The general conclusion was that ethanol at these doses caused no significant increase in oxygen consumption.
d   Alcoholic status not recorded.

microsomal enzyme induction would not be expected, and little change in oxygen consumption would be anticipated. For this same reason it is not unexpected that Lundquist et al. (1962b) reported no increase in the oxygen consumption of men with blood levels of ethanol apparently not exceeding 30mg per 100ml. Andersen et al. (1963) reported no increase in the metabolic rate of healthy young men given ethanol, but their subjects were purposely studied under cold conditions. In such a situation, the heat produced by microsomal metabolism would not be wasted, but would be usefully employed to reduce that required for thermogenic processes such as shivering. Hence no increase in metabolic rate would be predicted.

Animal studies concerning the effects of ethanol on oxygen consumption have produced conflicting results. Most of these studies have been complicated by a number of factors such as the opposing influences of sedation by ethanol and excitement associated with its forced administration. Many studies have shown a rise in oxygen consumption (Weiss and Reiss, 1923; Smythe et al., 1953; Heim et al., 1955; Perman, 1962b; Horvarth and Willard, 1962; Kalant et al., 1963) but in some there was no increase (Le Breton, 1936) or only a very delayed rise (Baron and Trémolières, 1968). It is of interest that an abnormal response of body weight to ethanol calories is not generally recognised despite the large number of studies in which ethanol has been given for prolonged periods of time. Wallgren and Barry (1970) have summarised these studies in table form. Unfortunately, pair feeding was not generally used, making it impossible to assess the efficiency of calorie utilization in most studies. Furthermore, total ethanol intakes were generally too low to saturate the MEOS

In vitro techniques involving rat livers have given conflicting results. Some authors reported that ethanol increased the oxygen consumption of tissue slices (Fondal and Kochakian, 1951) and of homogenates (Griffaton and Lowy, 1964), but others found no effect in tissue slices (Forsander, 1966) or in isolated perfused livers (Forsander et al., 1965). However, these data are difficult to assess because of probable incomplete saturation of MEOS in some experiments (Forsander, 1966; Griffaton and Lowy, 1964) and because the control values were markedly unstable (Forsander et al., 1965), or not relevant to the aim of the study and therefore not reported (Griffaton and Lowy, 1964).

6.10.4 Mechanisms of Wastage of Ethanol Calories: Alternative Possibilities

There are many possible ways whereby ethanol might produce metabolic inefficiency apart from those involving microsomal metabolism. However, there is little evidence that these are quantitatively significant. One possibility is that ethanol could increase the caloric losses in excreta, for example by producing malabsorption. However, the feeding of ethanol tends to actually decrease the faecal loss of fat (Rodrigo et al., 1971) or of nitrogen (Atwater and Benedict, 1896; Klatskin, 1961; Rodrigo et al., 1971). Of course, some ethanol is excreted unchanged, but measurements of total caloric losses in the excreta of rats, including losses in the breath showed that they were insufficient to account for the energy wastage produced by ethanol (Pirola and Lieber, 1975).

Ethanol could also stimulate other metabolic pathways that are not effectively coupled with phosphorylation to yield high-energy compounds. As discussed by Krebs (1960), calculations of the expected data suggest that the initial stages of amino acid degradation that prepare the molecule for entry into the citric acid cycle are not effectively coupled with ATP synthesis. Thus ethanol might conceivably enhance the body's energy requirements by stimulating inefficient pathways of protein metabolism or by increasing the overall rate of protein metabolism. In the latter situation, urinary nitrogen would be increased. However, the evidence that ethanol increases urinary nitrogen is conflicting (Atwater and Benedict, 1896; Shapiro, 1935; Mitchell, 1935; Rice et al., 1950; Summerskill et al., 1957; Klatskin, 1961; Trémolières et al., 1967; Rodrigo et al., 1971).

Another potential cause of energy wastage following ethanol ingestion is uncoupling of oxidative phosphorylation. This could result from the structural and functional changes produced in the hepatic mitochondria (Rubin et al., 1972) or it might result from stimulation of catecholamine secretion (Perman, 1961; Anton, 1965; Sobel et al., 1966). However, studies of a possible uncoupling effect of chronic ethanol ingestion have yielded conflicting results (Kiessling and Pillstrom, 1966; Banks et al., 1970; Toth et al., 1971).

Ethanol could also conceivably impair metabolic efficiency by directly increasing energy expenditure. Chronic ethanol intake in rats enhances the activity of Mg^{++} stimulated adenosine triphosphatase; the hepatic concentration of ATP falls and there is a rise in Pi (Walker and Gordon, 1970). Theoretically, this could have a significant effect on hepatic energy requirements. However, oxygen consumption under these conditions has not been determined. An increased expenditure of energy could also be required to replace the heat lost by vasodilatation associated with drinking alcohol. In this regard it is interesting to note that vasodilatation during drinking did not occur in subjects exposed to cold under carefully controlled conditions (Andersen et al., 1963). This raises the interesting possibility that vasodilatation during ethanol metabolism is partly a means of losing the excess heat produced during microsomal ethanol oxidation. This would be expected to occur only during drinking at comfortable environmental temperatures and would be abolished on exposure to cold. It is also interesting to note that in the above study, ethanol intake during cold exposure failed to produce a rise in the metabolic rate. Ethanol could also increase energy requirements if it increased muscular activity, but of course its sedative properties tend to have the reverse effect (Mitchell, 1935). Indeed, the failure of ethanol-fed rats to gain weight at the same rate as their pair-fed controls is all the more remarkable when one considers the tendency to a reduced physical activity of alcohol-fed animals. Ethanol increases the motility of the gut, at least under some experimental conditions (Pirola and Davis, 1970). However, experience with other dietary substances indicates that alimentary motor activity does not contribute significantly to total body oxygen requirements and appears to play no part in the specific dynamic action of protein (Wilhelmj et al., 1928).

6.10.5 Altered Energy Requirements with Drugs other than Ethanol

If energy wastage during chronic ethanol intake is partly due to increased hepatic microsomal enzyme activity, then one might anticipate that a similar metabolic inefficiency might be produced by other drugs capable of inducing microsomal enzymes. Of course the changes might be less marked because no other drug is metabolized at a rate comparable to the rate of ethanol oxidation. However, the metabolism of endogenous substrates by the endoplasmic reticulum would be expected to be markedly enhanced and this could also contribute to the loss of energy.

A number of animal experiments are compatible with this hypothesis, although by no means exclusively so (Pirola and Lieber, 1975, 1976). After receiving a standard dose of aminopyrine, oxygen consumption was 24% higher ($p < 0.01$) in rats pretreated with an 'inducing' course of phenobarbital than in saline-treated controls. In the absence of any drugs, 'induced' rats had a 6% higher ($p < 0.01$) oxygen consumption (fig. 14). The higher rate of metabolism in such animals was also shown by a 9% ($p < 0.05$) higher rate of weight loss when food and fluids were withdrawn. To exclude the possibility that such changes were due to agitation secondary to drug withdrawal, rats were also tested under anaesthesia. Under ethanol anaesthesia, oxygen consumption was 5% higher ($p < 0.01$) in animals previously fed an alcohol-containing diet than in pair-fed controls (fig. 15). Similarly, under hexobarbital anaesthesia, rats pretreated with an inducing course of phenobarbital had a 12% ($p < 0.001$) higher oxygen consumption than saline controls. In the latter experiment, varying doses of hexobarbital were used so that the comparisons of oxygen consumption could be made during anaesthesia of comparable depth. The metabolic rate of the whole body represents the net effect of innumerable biochemical and physiological

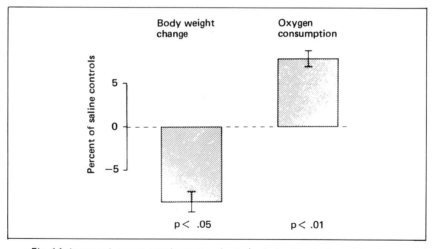

Fig. 14. Increased energy requirements of rats (as judged by body weight changes and O₂ consumption) after a four-day 'inducing' course of phenobarbital. In these experiments rats were tested 48 hours after the last dose of phenobarbital, i.e. during the metabolism of endogenous substrates.

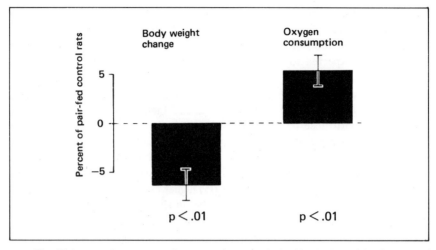

Fig. 15. Increased energy requirements of rats (as judged by body weight changes and
O$_2$ consumption) after chronic ethanol intake. Comparisons were made with pair-fed controls. Oxygen consumption was measured in 11 pairs under ethanol anaesthesia after 3—4
weeks of ethanol feeding. The changes in body weight were recorded during 15 days of
pair-feeding in 3 pairs.

reactions. A change after the administration of any one pharmacological agent
could be the result of any of a number of biological effects of that agent (as
discussed earlier in the case of ethanol). One factor common to all these experiments with their varied protocols, was the comparison between 'induced' and
'non-induced' animals. In each case, there was evidence of a higher metabolic
rate in the 'induced' animals. These findings support the concept that microsomal drug metabolism can impair the body's caloric balance. However, the full
evaluation of this hypothesis will have to await a number of further studies
involving many different drugs and employing different measurements of metabolic activity.

Weight watchers are traditionally advised to restrict their intake of alcoholic
beverages. This is sound general advice, but ironically, it may be less applicable
to those most likely to take alcohol and other drugs in excess. The combination
of inefficient pathways of microsomal drug metabolism and the effects of
induction of microsomal enzymes may alter the body's caloric requirements.
These effects could be of considerable significance to energy balance when a
major source of calories such as ethanol is being partly oxidized by hepatic
microsomes. Nutritional disturbances in alcoholism are common and result from
a variety of factors. The present hypothesis raises the possibility of a new
mechanism based on inefficient use of energy. Thus, to the extent that ethanol
abuse results in energy wastage, some calories of ethanol do not count.

7. Specific Alcohol-Drug Interactions

The general mechanisms underlying drug-alcohol interactions are summarised in section 1.4. Some of the better known examples are discussed below. The interactions have been classified according to their apparent involvement of the ADH and MEOS pathways. Obviously such a classification can never be completely satisfactory because of the complexity and variability of most drug interactions and the fact that many mechanisms may be involved. Not all the interactions are undesirable. For example the interactions with ethylene glycol and methanol have therapeutic applications. The list of drugs discussed here is by no means exhaustive, and for a more complete summary, the reader is referred to the annotated bibliography published by the Addiction Research Foundation of Ontario, Canada (Polacsek et al., 1972) or to the detailed reviews by Wallgren and Barry (1970) and Kissin (1974b).

7.1 Interactions Largely Involving the ADH Pathway

7.1.1 Ethylene Glycol

Ethylene glycol is widely used industrially as a solvent and in hydraulic systems, and as an anti-freeze solution for automobile radiators. It is a central nervous system depressant that causes an intoxication similar to that produced by ethanol. The fatal dose is approximately 100g.

Ethylene glycol is oxidized by ADH to its corresponding aldehyde (von Wartburg et al., 1964) and then to oxalic acid. The latter is toxic to the brain and kidneys; calcium oxalate crystals are deposited in nervous and renal tissues and the serum calcium may fall (Dreisbach, 1963). Hepatic and myocardial damage are also seen. Three stages may be recognised clinically (Morini, 1954). Initially there is an intoxication similar to acute alcoholism. Within a few hours, vomiting, signs of cardiac failure and deepening coma are seen. If the patient survives 24 hours or more, cyanosis, psychological disturbances and acute renal failure appear. Thus death may occur from respiratory depression within the first few hours or from pulmonary oedema or renal failure after one or two days.

Ethanol has been found to be effective therapy (Wacker et al., 1965). It competitively inhibits ethylene glycol oxidation, so that the compound is gradually excreted unchanged. Other therapeutic measures include the administration of calcium gluconate to precipitate oxalic acid, and general and emergency measures such as gastric lavage and treatment of respiratory depression, pulmonary oedema and renal failure.

7.1.2 Disulfiram (Antabuse)

Tetraethylthiuram disulphide (TETD, disulfiram, Antabuse) is used in the rubber industry, and workers exposed to it were noted to develop an abnormal reaction to alcohol (Jacobsen, 1950). Previously, Williams (1937) noted that industrial exposure to tetramethylthiuram disulphide (TMTD) caused a hypersensitivity to ethanol and he suggested that this effect might be useful in the treatment of alcoholism. But the main interest in the therapeutic use of disulfiram began when two Danish physicians took the drug during an investigation of its antihelminthic properties and subsequently became ill at a cocktail party (Hald and Jacobsen, 1948a, 1948b).

The disulfiram-ethanol reaction begins within 5–10 minutes of ethanol ingestion with marked peripheral vasodilatation, starting in the face, intense throbbing in the head and neck, throbbing headache, vomiting, dyspnoea, chest pain, sweating, thirst, confusion and hypotension. Mild reactions may be elicited by as little as 7ml and last 30 minutes. Severe reactions may last several hours. Complete recovery is the rule but death may occur, preceded by pallor and shock.

The therapeutic value of disulfiram in alcoholism is very limited. It is not a cure, but it can be taken by the patient who wants to strengthen his resolve by knowing that he cannot take alcohol for at least three or four days after taking disulfiram. The full co-operation of the patient is vital to avoid potentially fatal reactions to unusual sources of ethanol such as cough syrups, sauces, fermented vinegar and fruit juices, and the drug should be given only under medical supervision. Because of the potential danger of disulfiram therapy, there has been a search for similar drugs with less dramatic effects. The use of citrated calcium carbimide (Temposil) has been suggested (Ferguson, 1956). The duration of action is shorter (Mitchell, 1958) and the circulatory changes are less severe than after taking disulfiram (Marconi et al., 1961).

The disulfiram-ethanol reaction is sometimes referred to as the acetaldehyde reaction because its severity correlates with the blood acetaldehyde level (Hine et al., 1952; Raby, 1954) and many of its features can be reproduced by infusion of acetaldehyde (Asmussen et al., 1948). Using enzymatic and radio-isotopic methods respectively, Wagner (1957) and Casier and Polet (1958) expressed doubts concerning the presence of elevated acetaldehyde levels after disulfiram and ethanol. However, a review of 25 reports involving 7 species (Truitt and Walsh, 1971) and including gas chromatographic studies (Truitt and Duritz, 1966; Walsh and Truitt, 1968) shows that most authors found several-fold greater rises in blood acetaldehyde after ethanol and disulfiram than after ethanol alone. The rise in blood acetaldehyde is due to inhibition of aldehyde dehydrogenase, apparently through competition with NAD for the active centres of the enzyme.

However, acetaldehyde normally has an adrenergic vasoconstrictor action. Thus some features of the ethanol – disulfiram reaction, notably the vasodilatation and hypotension, cannot be explained solely on the basis of acetaldehyde accumulation and other possible explanations have been sought (Wagner, 1957; Perman, 1962c; Casier and Merlevede, 1962; Forney and Harger, 1969). Truitt and Walsh (1971) have summarised the evidence in favour of their hypothesis that there are four components to the ethanol-disulfiram reaction:

1) disulfiram inhibits aldehyde dehydrogenase, causing increased levels of acetaldehyde

2) increased levels of acetaldehyde cause release of norepinephrine, evoking a transient vasoconstrictive action (Akabane et al., 1964; Walsh and Truitt, 1968)

3) disulfiram blocks dopamine-β-oxidase, lowering the norepinephrine content of tissues and preventing resynthesis of norepinephrine (Musacchio et al., 1966; Thoenen et al., 1967)

4) with norepinephrine depleted, the hypotension and vasodilatation can be produced by the direct depressant action of acetaldehyde on the myocardium and smooth muscle of blood vessels (James and Bear, 1967, 1968; Walsh et al., 1969).

An abnormal response to ethanol similar to the disulfiram-ethanol reaction can also occur in a number of other situations, including industrial exposure to cyanamide (Hald et al., 1952), eating the fungus Coprinus atramentarius (Fisher, 1945) and ingestion of animal charcoal (Clark and Hulpieu, 1958b). Drugs that have some disulfiram-like activity include the hypoglycaemic sulphonylureas (Truitt et al., 1962), the anti-parasitic agent, metronidazole (Flagyl) (Lal, 1969) and an antimicrobial drug, furazolidine (Perman, 1965).

7.2 Interactions Largely Involving MEOS

7.2.1 Barbiturates

The increased tolerance of the alcoholic to sedative and anaesthetic agents is common knowledge. This has been most intensively studied in the case of the barbiturates, but involves also the phenothiazines, meprobamate, chloral hydrate and anaesthetic agents. Some form of pharmacodynamic tolerance is involved since at the same blood levels, animals tolerant to barbiturates and alcohol show less sedation than non-tolerant animals. However, the differences in CNS depression become less with increasing blood levels so that the lethal blood concentration for these drugs is not very much elevated (Jaffe, 1970). This puts the alcoholic and habitual drug taker in the dangerous situation of having a reduced margin between the therapeutic and lethal blood concentrations of sedatives. For this reason alone, the barbiturates are best avoided in the treatment of delirium tremens, especially when one considers that these drugs themselves are addicting. Furthermore, other effective agents such as diazepam (Valium) and chlordiazepoxide (Librium) are available for the treatment of delirium tremens (Greenblatt and Greenblatt, 1972).

Ethanol also interacts with a number of barbiturates at a microsomal level (see section 5.4.3). When the barbiturate is taken with ethanol, the metabolism of each is inhibited, resulting in higher blood levels and slower clearance. Thus it is not surprising that fatalities have been reported (Swidler, 1971). Mould et al. (1972) reported that the blood ethanol after glutethimide and ethanol was 30 per cent higher than after ethanol alone. This was reflected in impaired reaction times. By contrast, the alcoholic when sober has an accelerated rate of drug metabolism in the hepatic smooth endoplasmic reticulum, thus providing him with an increased metabolic drug tolerance. Thus Misra et al. (1971) found that feeding ethanol for four weeks reduced the half-life of pentobarbital by 25%.

7.2.2 Anticonvulsants

Most anticonvulsant drugs are metabolized by the hepatic smooth endoplasmic reticulum so that much of what has been said about sedatives such as phenobarbital, applies equally to this group of drugs. Thus the metabolism of diphenylhydantoin (Dilantin) is accelerated in the alcoholic (Kater et al., 1969). In addition, alcoholism itself may contribute to the development of seizures, especially during acute withdrawal, making adequate drug therapy difficult. Folic acid deficiency is also a common complication of alcoholism and could enhance the tendency to folic acid depletion that occurs in patients receiving diphenylhydantoin. The mechanism of folic acid depletion complicating anti-convulsant therapy is unknown. An early view was that there was interference with absorption of folic acid but evidence for this is conflicting (Reynolds, 1972). Another possibility is that hepatic microsomal enzyme induction results in an increased rate of metabolism of folate (Maxwell et al., 1972). In support of this view, Latham et al. (1973) reported that of four anticonvulsants tested, pheneturide was a more potent inducer of hepatic microsomal enzymes than phenobarbitone, phenytoin or primidone, and that pheneturide was also associated with the greatest reduction in serum folate levels. If this view is correct, then ethanol-induced microsomal changes may also contribute to the folic acid deficiency of alcoholics in addition to such recognised factors as poor dietary intake, malabsorption and liver disease (Vitale and Coffey, 1971). Whatever the mechanism of folate depletion, it could aggravate the tendency of anticon-vulsants to produce megaloblastic anaemia. For reasons unknown, folic acid deficiency can also enhance the effectiveness of these drugs in controlling seizures. However, this marginal benefit should in no way override the estab-lished view that abstention from alcohol is desirable in epileptics.

7.2.3 Meprobamate

Meprobamate is an anxiety reducing agent of doubtful value with a high potential for the development of dependence and drug abuse (Isbell and Chrúsciel, 1970). It has a synergistic depressant effect on performance tasks in humans when given with ethanol (Goldberg, 1970). This appears to be largely due to interference with microsomal drug metabolism. Thus Rubin et al. (1970b) found that ethanol reduced the rate of meprobamate metabolism by rat liver slices. The clinical significance of this *in vitro* effect was shown by two- to five-fold increases in the half-life of meprobamate in non-alcoholic volunteers given ethanol. By contrast, the chronic administration of ethanol produced a metabolic tolerance to meprobamate (Misra et al., 1971). This is similar to that which develops with the barbiturates and is due to hepatic microsomal enzyme induction. The half-life of meprobamate in non-alcoholic volunteers was halved by four weeks of high ethanol intake (Misra et al., 1971).

7.2.4 Tricyclic Antidepressants

In the last few years there has been widespread use of these drugs in the treatment of depression, notwithstanding the fact that their mechanism of action is as uncertain as is the pathogenesis of the conditions for which they are prescribed. They tend to have both sedative and depressant effects on the central nervous system. Included in this group of drugs are imipramine (Tofranil), amitriptyline (Tryptanol), desipramine (Norpramin, Pertofrane), nortriptyline (Aventyl) and protriptyline (Vivactyl). Their detoxification generally involves phase I and phase II reactions in the liver so that, as in the case of the barbiturates, one might anticipate that ingestion with alcohol acutely could cause decreased drug tolerance whereas chronic alcohol consumption could enhance drug tolerance. It should also be borne in mind that the antidepressant actions take several days to develop fully and that sedation may be a problem in the first few days of therapy. This applies more to normal subjects than to patients with psychotic depression.

Apart from interactions with ethanol at the hepatic level (altered metabolic tolerance) there may be changes in pharmacological tolerance. This depends on the ratio of sedative to stimulant activity of the drug in question. In reviewing this, Kissin (1974b) concluded that the tricyclic antidepressants could be either synergistic or antagonistic to ethanol according to their ratio of sedative/ stimulant activity. Using this criterion, the drugs could be listed in the following order: amitriptyline, trimipramine, imipramine, nortriptyline, protriptyline and desipramine. Amitriptyline is the most sedative of the drugs and is the most potentiating to ethanol. Desipramine is the most stimulant and is the most antagonistic to ethanol.

Patients taking tricyclic antidepressants should be cautioned against alcohol, especially during the early stages of therapy. A number of fatalities have been reported (Lockett and Milner, 1965; Milner, 1967; Steel et al., 1967; Fuge, 1967; Masters, 1967). In two of these cases, only standard therapeutic doses of amitriptyline appeared to have been taken, the blood concentrations of ethanol were not remarkable, and no other drugs were known to have been ingested (Lockett and Milner, 1965). Thus it is not surprising that the combination of these drugs with alcohol intake adversely affects motor skills such as those involved in driving (Landauer et al., 1969). It is conceivable that this contributes to a number of sudden deaths otherwise classed as being due to motor accidents, drowning or of unknown cause.

7.2.5 Anticoagulants

The safe and effective use of oral anticoagulants can be difficult at the best of times, but the difficulties are undoubtedly compounded in the alcoholic. This is not surprising when one considers that most of the coagulation factors are produced in the liver, that the prothrombin time can be altered by dietary changes, especially malnutrition and that oral anticoagulants are metabolized by the hepatic smooth endoplasmic reticulum.

Drinking alcohol alone (in the form of whisky or wine) was reported by Riedler (1966) to affect the blood levels of coagulation factors. He found an initial transient increase followed by a subsequent decrease. Probably more important is the fact that oral anticoagulants are detoxified by microsomal enzyme pathways. This provides the basis for the well known interference of other drugs in therapy with coumarin derivatives (Formiller and Cohon, 1969). Patients admitted to hospital for acute alcoholism show a significantly accelerated clearance of warfarin (Kater et al., 1969). Thus to achieve the same level of anticoagulation, such patients will require a higher dose of warfarin than nondrinking patients. Furthermore, this increased requirement would not be stable and might be expected to fall after admission to hospital and withdrawal of alcohol.

7.2.6 Carbon Tetrachloride

Carbon tetrachloride is widely used as a solvent and cleaning agent (especially in dry cleaning) and in fire extinguishers. Acute poisoning may follow ingestion, inhalation or absorption through the skin. Early features are abdominal pain, vomiting, hypotension and depression of the central nervous system. If the patient survives the initial coma, clinical evidence of hepatic and/or renal failure may develop within a few days. However, biochemical evidence of early hepatic damage can be shown to occur within 30 minutes of CCl_4 administration (Recknagel, 1967).

It has long been known that the toxicity of carbon tetrachloride is aggravated by alcohol (Smillie and Pessoa, 1923; Polacsek et al., 1972). Dreisbach (1963) recommended that workers using CCl_4 should not drink alcoholic beverages. However, it is only recently that advances have been made in elucidating the mechanism of this potentiation (Hasumura et al., 1974). It had been suggested that ethanol might enhance CCl_4 absorption from the gastrointestinal tract (Klatskin, 1969), but Cornish and Adefuin (1966) reported that hepatic damage occurred when CCl_4 was given by inhalation and could still occur 15 hours after ethanol withdrawal. It is now generally accepted that the major toxicity of CCl_4 is due to its metabolites which are formed during interaction with hepatic microsomal mixed function oxidases (Recknagel, 1967). These metabolites appear to produce damage by irreversible binding to microsomal protein and lipid. Thus induction of hepatic microsomal enzymes by phenobarbital enhances CCl_4 toxicity (Garner and McLean, 1969). Hasumura et al. (1974) have shown that a similar mechanism, namely microsomal enzyme induction, is responsible for the enhanced CCl_4 toxicity produced by ethanol. These authors reported that rats chronically fed ethanol had an increased covalent binding of $^{14}CCl_4$ metabolites to microsomal protein in vitro. Furthermore, hepatic microsomes from these rats showed greater *in vitro* destruction of cyto-chrome P-450 by CCl_4 than did microsomes from control animals. The micro-somal metabolism of $^{14}CCl_4$ to $^{14}CO_2$ *in vitro* was also enhanced by prior ethanol feeding and the greater hepatic damage *in vivo* was not dependent on the presence of ethanol at the time of CCl_4 administration.

7.3 Interactions Involving Both ADH and MEOS

7.3.1 Phenothiazines

Therapeutic doses of antipsychotic drugs cause some degree of central nervous system depression and potentiate that produced by ethanol (Zirkle et al., 1959; Berger, 1969). In an earlier monograph in this series, Milner (1972) reported on the effects of combinations of ethanol and psychotropic drugs on driving. He concluded that in general, the greater the usual sedative activity of the drug, the greater the risk of its adding to the adverse effects of alcohol on driving. He also suggested that a change in prescribing habits might be used for selected patients to reduce the hazards of such activities as driving while main-taining an effective antianxiety regimen. The hypnotic effects of drugs such as chlorpromazine, thioridazine and doxepin could be turned to advantage to achieve a sedative effect at night and a residual antianxiety response through the next day. Thus a heavy evening dose with 1 or 2 small doses during the day will still permit an antidepressant effect to develop during a course of therapy. Meanwhile, the hazards of complex daily activities would be reduced.

The mechanism of chlorpromazine-ethanol reactions is uncertain. A direct sensory attenuation seems likely. In addition, chlorpromazine may affect the rate of ethanol absorption (see section 2.2.5). Impaired activity of ADH may also be a factor, but the evidence for this is not strong. *In vitro* studies show that chlorpromazine produces a non-competitive inhibition of horse liver ADH (Khouw et al., 1963). However, *in vivo* studies have shown no effect of chlor-promazine on ethanol clearance in man (Casier et al., 1966) and little or no effect in animals (Seidel and Soehring, 1965; Smith et al., 1961). The dis-tribution of ethanol may also be affected by chlorpromazine. Some investigators have reported a highly erratic descending limb of the blood alcohol curve after chlorpromazine and Kalant (1971) postulated that this was due to fluctuations in peripheral blood flow, especially through skeletal muscle and skin, rather than to variations in the rate of metabolism. Finally, both ethanol and the pheno-thiazines are partly metabolized by the hepatic smooth endoplasmic reticulum and could thus interact at a microsomal level. The principal metabolic pathway of chlorpromazine is hydroxylation and subsequent conjugation to form a glucuronide. Phenothiazines also undergo demethylation reactions or may be excreted as sulphoxides. Thus, as discussed in connection with phenobarbital in sections 6.7, 6.8, the acute administration of ethanol together with a phenothiazine might result in competitive inhibition in the smooth endoplasmic reticulum with decreased clearance of one or both drugs and enhanced sedative effects. By contrast, a phenothiazine given alone to an alcoholic with an enhanced activity of smooth endoplasmic reticulum might be cleared very rapidly resulting in a reduced sedative effect. However, if the alcoholism were severe, the sedative effect could be enhanced as a result of hepatic decompensation (and impaired microsomal enzyme function) or hepatic precoma (with an increased sensitivity of the brain to various drugs).

7.3.2 Hypoglycaemic Agents

Ethanol alone causes disturbances of carbohydrate metabolism that are of special relevance to the diabetic (Arky, 1971). Alcohol ingestion can cause a profound and dangerous hypoglycaemia in a patient with absent glycogen stores. The latter may result from fasting such as may occur during an acute illness or in association with an alcoholic debauch or alcoholic gastritis and it may be enhanced by an underlying endocrine disorder such as hyperthyroidism or adrenocortical insufficiency. Ethanol metabolism also impairs gluconeogenesis at a number of levels as a result of the reduced NAD/NADH ratio secondary to alcohol dehydrogenase activity (fig. 16). The oxidation of glycerophosphate and of lactate is impaired, citric acid cycle activity is strikingly reduced and entrance of glutamate into the citric acid cycle (a major link between protein and carbohydrate metabolism) is inhibited. Availability of acetyl Co A is also reduced. This compound is an activator of the enzyme catalyzing the conversion of pyruvate to oxaloacetate, a reaction that plays a major part in controlling gluconeogenesis. Changes in the cytosolic NAD/NADH ratio also cause a rise in serum levels of lactic acid and ketones (Lieber et al., 1971).

Alcohol can create severe clinical problems in diabetics in a number of ways. The sulphonylurea compounds stimulate the pancreatic release of insulin and the latter inhibits hepatic gluconeogenesis and glucose output. These effects are augmented in the presence of ethanol. The latter may also impair the judgement of the diabetic and lead to errors in dosage of medication or assessment of caloric intake. A severe and prolonged hypoglycaemia can result with irreversible neurological damage (Arky et al., 1968). Rarely, the sulphonylureas can induce a disulfiram-like reaction in the presence of ethanol (Truitt et al., 1962). The effect is most likely to occur with chlorpropamide and appears to involve inhibition of acetaldehyde activity (Podgainy and Bressler, 1968). A less dramatic but more common complication of alcohol is the induction of hepatic microsomal pathways responsible for drug metabolism. This produces a significantly

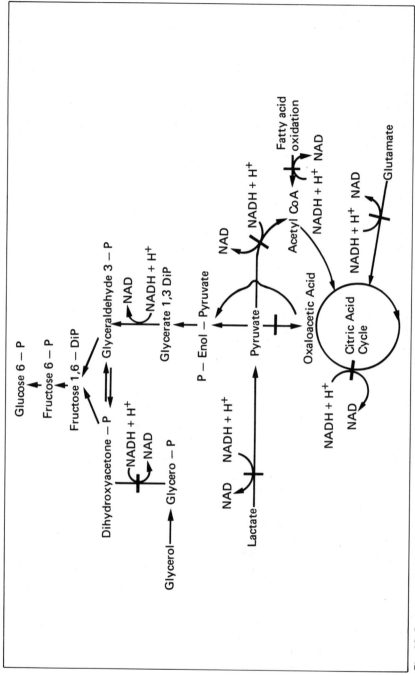

Fig. 16. Pathways of gluconeogenesis showing reactions that may be inhibited by a raised NADH/NAD ratio secondary to ethanol oxidation.

increased drug tolerance to the sulphonylureas as shown by reduction in the half-life of tolbutamide (Kater et al., 1969c; Carulli et al., 1971).

The biguanide compound, phenformin, is widely used in the treatment of maturity-onset diabetes, and as an adjunct to 'smooth' the response to insulin in some 'unstable' diabetics. Its mechanism of action is unknown. It has been implicated in the production of lactic acidosis in diabetes, although it is difficult to exclude associated renal or cardiovascular disease as the major factor in these cases. Ethanol ingestion preceded symptoms in several cases of lactic acidosis associated with phenformin therapy (Davidson et al., 1966). In non-diabetic volunteers, phenformin, like ethanol, raises the serum lactate concentration as a result of enhanced production and decreased utilization; it also antagonizes the inhibitory effect of ethanol on gluconeogenesis from lactate (Kreisberg et al., 1972).

The use (and especially the abuse) of alcoholic beverages can give rise to problems in the management of diabetes in a number of other ways. The calorie content of alcoholic drinks has to be accounted for in the dietary calculations of diabetics. Chronic alcoholism may be associated with neglect of diet, predisposition to trauma and infection and failure to take medications in the prescribed manner. The symptoms of acute alcoholism may mask those of hypoglycaemia or of diabetic ketosis. Chronic pancreatic insufficiency punctuated by episodes of acute pancreatic inflammation may develop and these may affect insulin secretion. Acute ethanol ingestion may cause catecholamine release, leading to hyperglycaemia (Lieber, 1972b). Glucose intolerance may also be partly due to decreased peripheral glucose utilization, possibly as a result of ethanol-induced ketosis (Lieber, 1973b).

7.3.3 Chloral Hydrate

The famous 'Micky Finn' effect is the result of enhanced sedation produced by chloral hydrate when taken in the presence of ethanol. However, this reaction seems to have been exaggerated in folklore. It is probably partly due to a direct additive effect on the central nervous system similar to that produced by a combination of alcohol with most sedatives. In addition there are metabolic interactions between ethanol and chloral hydrate.

The main hypnotic effect following chloral hydrate ingestion is thought to be due to its metabolic product trichloroethanol. The two agents have comparable sedative properties (Owens et al., 1955), but the conversion of the former to the latter is so rapid that it is difficult to detect chloral hydrate in body fluids after ingestion of therapeutic doses (Marshall and Owens, 1954). The reaction is catalyzed by ADH with NADH as cofactor (Friedman and Cooper, 1960). Part of the trichloroethanol is conjugated and excreted as a glucuronide.

Chloral hydrate can also be converted to the inactive trichloroacetic acid by an enzyme system with NAD as cofactor (Cooper and Friedman, 1958). Thus ethanol oxidation by the ADH pathway with its associated decreased NAD/NADH ratio would simultaneously favour formation of the inactive metabolite trichloroacetic acid. Also, small concentrations of trichloroethanol are known to inhibit ethanol oxidation by hepatic homogenates (Friedman and Cooper, 1960). However, the relevance of these metabolic relationships to the enhanced sedative effect seen clinically is uncertain. Kaplan et al. (1967a) found no difference in the elimination rates of chloral hydrate and ethanol when given singly or in combination to humans, while in mice, conflicting results have been obtained (Kaplan et al., 1967b; Gessner and Dien, 1969; Cabana and Gessner, 1970).

It is possible that other pathways of chloral hydrate metabolism are concerned in the enhanced sedation produced by simultaneous alcohol intake. Excretion as trichloroethanol (or its glucuronide) and trichloroacetic acid does not account for the dose of chloral hydrate ingested (Marshall and Owens, 1954; Owens and Marshall, 1955). The possible importance of microsomal enzymes is suggested by the observation that the metabolism of coumarin anticoagulants is affected by chloral hydrate therapy (Cucinell et al., 1966). Thus ethanol might conceivably affect the metabolism of chloral hydrate in much the same way as it affects the degradation of phenobarbital, the net clinical effect of the drugs depending, in part, on the duration of administration and whether or not they are given simultaneously (see sections 6.7, 6.8).

7.3.4 Methanol

Methanol poisoning is a medical emergency. Toxicity correlates poorly with the dose; 70 to 100ml are usually fatal although death has been reported after as little as 5ml (Closs, 1971). The main features are:

1) early and severe acidosis,

2) a specific retinal toxicity that becomes evident 6 to 48 hours after ingestion,

3) depression of the central nervous system (Ritchie, 1970; Closs, 1971).

The conversion of methanol to formaldehyde can be accomplished *in vitro* by ADH (Blair and Vallee, 1966; Makar et al., 1968), the microsomal alcohol oxidizing system (Lieber and De Carli, 1970a) and catalase (Tephly et al., 1964). However, it is likely that *in vivo* ADH and catalase are unimportant. ADH has a low affinity for methanol and is probably only active at concentrations causing death from toxicity of the central nervous system. A large number of enzymes can convert formaldehyde to formic acid, including aldehyde dehydrogenase, xanthine oxidase, aldehyde oxidase, glyceraldehyde-3-phosphate dehydrogenase, catalase, peroxidase and formate dehydrogenase (Cooper and Kini, 1962). The mechanism of the acidosis is uncertain but acids other than formic acid are mainly involved (Harrop and Benedict, 1920; Van Slyke and Palmer, 1920). The retinal damage appears to result from a product of methanol metabolism, possibly formaldehyde, the effect of which is aggravated by acidosis (Mardones, 1963). Early clinical features are headache, vertigo, vomiting and abdominal and back pain. Serious prognostic findings are visual disturbances, bradycardia and coma. Blindness usually precedes death, and coma and death may occur suddenly (Bennett et al., 1953). Restlessness and delirium are common. Hypotension is uncommon, and despite the acidosis, Kussmaul respiration is unusual. Laboratory findings include severe acidosis with comparatively mild ketosis, the presence in blood and urine of methanol in the early stages and formic acid in the later stages, and hyperamylasaemia due to pancreatitis.

The main points in therapy are prompt correction of acidosis and the administration of ethanol. Because methanol is oxidised at a rate of about one seventh of that for ethanol, total elimination from the body may take up to four days and therapy has to be correspondingly prolonged. Selected cases will require dialysis (Humphrey, 1974). It is important to take advantage of the lag period in the appearance of retinal and other neurological signs to forestall their appearance. The therapeutic value of ethanol was first noted by an anonymous U.S. army surgeon and reported by Bullar and Wood (1904). It was subsequently rediscovered by Roe (1943). Ethanol competitively inhibits methanol metabolism. A dose sufficient to keep the level of ethanol in the blood between 100 and 150mg per 100ml is recommended. Care should be taken when giving ethanol during therapy for the correction of acidosis because the sudden block in methanol oxidation will reduce the formation of organic acids with a danger of iatrogenic alkalosis.

7.4 Miscellaneous

7.4.1 Monoamine Oxidase (MAO) Inhibitors

This is a rather heterogeneous group of drugs that have in common the ability to block the oxidative deamination of biogenic amines. The relationship between this action and the therapeutic usefulness of these agents is uncertain. Included in this group of drugs are tranylcypromine (Parnate), phenelzine (Nardil), isocarboxazid (Marplan), nialamide (Niamide) and pargyline (Eutonyl).

The main effects appear to be on hepatic enzymes and are not specific for monoamine oxidase. A number of other oxidative reactions are also affected, resulting in impaired metabolism of various drugs, including ethanol, barbiturates, and aminopyrine (Jarvik, 1970). It should be borne in mind that effective antidepressant action may take weeks to appear. By contrast, the acute toxic effects of overdosage appear within hours of starting therapy, as does the interference with the metabolism of other drugs. Thus in the early stages of therapy, the patient may be at increased risk from suicidal tendencies associated with the depression.

However, the most dramatic complication of therapy with the MAO inhibitors is the hypertensive crisis (Beckman, 1967). This resembles the reaction seen in patients with phaeochromocytoma. There is usually severe headache, fever, an alarming elevation of blood pressure, and cardiac arrhythmias and intracranial bleeding may occur. The reaction may be fatal. It may follow the concomitant administration of drugs such as sympathomimetic amines, methyldopa, dopamine, and tryptophan or may be associated with the ingestion of certain alcoholic beverages and foods. The reaction is due to the presence of agents such as tyramine and dihydroxyphenylalanine (DOPA) in the foods. Tyramine is a pressor amine that releases norepinephrine from the tissues. In the presence of MAO inhibitors, the degradation of tyramine is blocked and the enhanced tissue level of tyramine results in greater release of norepinephrine which has also accumulated at nerve endings. DOPA is a precursor of dopamine and its accumulation produces effects similar to those produced by tyramine.

Dietary components that have been specially implicated because of their content of tyramine include beer, wine, most cheeses, canned figs and yeast products. Foods containing DOPA include beer, broad beans and yoghurt. Bananas should be avoided because of their serotonin content while the factors responsible for the precipitation of adverse reactions with chicken liver and pickled herring are uncertain. Not all alcoholic drinks have been implicated in hypertensive reactions with MAO inhibitors. However, because of the variability in the non-ethanol components of alcoholic beverages and in order to avoid confusion on the part of patients receiving these drugs, they should be advised against taking alcoholic drinks at all. It should also be noted that enzyme inhibition by these agents is irreversible. Return of monoamine oxidase activity depends on enzyme regeneration, a process which is not completely effective for weeks after stopping therapy. In this time, the risks of hypertensive crisis will continue, a point that should be emphasised to the patient.

7.4.2 Benzodiazepines

These are effective anxiety agents with a high safety index and a low potential for the development of dependence and drug abuse (Isbell and Chrúsciel, 1970). The group includes chlordiazepoxide (Librium) and diazepam (Valium). They contrast with meprobamate in that they have very little additive effect with ethanol and in most studies were found to actually antagonize it (see

Kissin, 1974b). The mechanism of this antagonism is unknown. These agents are effective in the treatment of acute ethanol withdrawal (Greenblatt and Greenblatt, 1972) and are possibly the anti-anxiety agent of choice for most alcoholics and in most stages of their illness.

7.4.3 Morphine and Related Drugs

There is no demonstrable cross tolerance between ethanol and morphine or its derivatives (i.e. individuals with increased tolerance to ethanol do not have enhanced tolerance to morphine). This contrasts with the cross tolerance between ethanol and many other hypnotics such as the barbiturates, chloral hydrate and paraldehyde. Thus the neuropharmacological effects of ethanol and morphine may involve basically different mechanisms. This is supported by the differences in the clinical features of acute intoxication (and withdrawal) of morphine and ethanol.

Ethanol and morphine actually have a potentiating effect on one another. This is exemplified by a number of reported deaths in alcoholics. However, the mechanism of this potentiation is unknown. It would appear that the repeated intake of ethanol sensitizes the brain to the effects of morphine in some way that is independent of the actual presence of ethanol. Thus, the pretreatment of mice with ethanol increases their mortality after morphine even when the latter drug is given after blood alcohol levels are undetectable (Venho et al., 1955). Of particular interest is a syndrome reported by Roizin (1969) in patients on a methadone maintenance programme for heroin withdrawal. Such patients have a high predisposition to secondary alcohol addiction. This in turn predisposes them to a syndrome with a high mortality characterised by fever and jaundice and rapidly terminating with coma and death. Autopsy shows an acute encephalopathy (mainly of the midbrain) and acute alcoholic hepatitis. The former appears to be related to the methadone treatment or heroin addiction since it is not seen in other cases of fatal alcoholic hepatitis. Roizin (1969) showed that there was disruption of catecholamine secreting cells in the midbrain and concluded that the syndrome represented a disturbance of catecholamine metabolism.

7.4.4 Amphetamines

The physiological and psychomotor interactions between ethanol and the amphetamines have been reviewed by Kissin (1974b). In many physiological studies, these drugs act as true antagonists, as judged by the effects of amphetamines on such indicators as recovery time after anaesthetising doses of ethanol, and ethanol induced nystagmus and changes in the electroencephalogram. However, the disinhibiting effect of ethanol that is seen early in acute intoxication potentiates the excitability produced by the amphetamines. Thus the drugs may be both antagonistic or synergistic in their physiological responses, depending on the type of response being produced by ethanol. The effects of a combination of these drugs on psychomotor performance is difficult to assess. A number of studies have yielded conflicting results. It would seem that the interaction of the two drugs is more complex than could be explained by a simple depressant/stimulant antagonism.

7.4.5 Caffeine

Caffeine and ethanol are antagonists. Generally speaking, ethanol impairs psychomotor performance; caffeine improves it. Thus there is some theoretical basis for the widely expressed view that the drive home after a party will be safer if it is preceded by a cup of coffee. Unfortunately, experimental studies do not support this contention (Forney and Hughes, 1970). Numerous studies have yielded conflicting results. This may be partly due to altered rates of absorption (see section 2.2.5) or it may be that the effects of caffeine will vary according to whether the depressant or excitatory effects of ethanol are predominant (as in the case of the amphetamines). However, caffeine is a weaker stimulant than the amphetamines so that any antagonism or synergism that is produced is probably of no practical significance.

7.4.6 β-Adrenergic Blocking Agents

An interesting modification of the effects of ethanol is that produced by the β-adrenergic blocking agent propranolol (see Kissin, 1974b). It produces an antiethanol effect by inhibiting the adrenergic system that accounts for the euphoriant effects of ethanol. It has the advantage that, unlike the amphetamines, it is itself a sedative. Carlsson and Johannson (1971) found it to be effective in the treatment of alcoholics both during acute toxicity and acute withdrawal. Others have found that it reduced the euphoriant effect of alcohol in alcoholics and that it reduced the preference for alcohol of conditioned monkeys (Kissin, 1947b).

7.4.7 Salicylates

Any effects of ethanol on salicylate excretion would be of interest because of the widespread self-administration of these compounds. Furthermore the salicylates compete with a large number of other compounds for conjugation to sulphates and glucuronides. Thus, any agent prolonging the elevation of the plasma salicylate level might delay the inactivation of other prescribed compounds such as isoproterenol and thyroxine. However, ethanol alone does not appear to affect salicylate elimination (Levy, 1971). The main mechanism of salicylate excretion is the urinary passage of the glycine conjugate, salicylurate. The hepatic synthesis of the latter is the rate-limiting step. It is at least of some theoretical interest that giving ethanol reduces salicylate excretion if sodium benzoate is administered at the same time. Benzoate is an inhibitor of salicylurate formation and products containing both salicylate and p-aminobenzoic acid are marketed with the intention of prolonging the action of the salicylate. Ethanol reduces the conjugation of benzoate to hippuric acid. Thus the administration of ethanol with benzoate aggravates the reduction in the rate of salicylurate formation that is produced by benzoate alone (Levy, 1971).

7.4.8 Chlormethiazole (Hemineurin)

This drug is a sedative and anticonvulsant that is chemically related to the thiazole portion of the vitamin B_1 molecule. Its value in the treatment of acute alcohol withdrawal is well established, and it is now widely used in hospital practice. Its effectiveness may be partly due to the normalization of urinary catecholamine levels. Because of its potency and the fact that dependence on the drug itself may develop, it is best used in short courses in hospitalised patients. When taken with alcohol, depression of the central nervous system is enhanced. The exact mechanisms responsible remain to be determined, but are probably similar to those discussed in the case of the barbiturates. There is probably both a direct additive effect and a competitive inhibition at an hepatic microsomal level.

8. The Congeners of Alcoholic Beverages

Ethanol is the main physiologically active component of most alcoholic beverages. Together with water it comprises the greater part of alcoholic drinks. The remaining fraction is made up by the congeners. Their concentrations in various alcoholic beverages are summarised in tables XII, XIII, XIV. Although quantitatively small, they play a crucial and often overlooked role in the social use and abuse of alcoholic beverages. It is the seemingly minor variations on congener content that enable us to distinguish the bouquet of a Hunter River claret from a Barossa Valley burgundy. Thus the congener content, and the factors modifying it are a subject of considerable interest to the wine, beer and spirits industries (Amerine, 1966; Leake and Silverman, 1966, 1971). They are also of particular interest to historians, because the story of alcohol consumption over the centuries is closely intertwined with the development of cultural patterns and the social changes of different civilizations (Leake and Silverman, 1966). An understanding of these variations in drinking patterns and their associated social changes are of importance in the study and treatment of alcoholism.

The congeners are often highly volatile compounds comprising mainly a variety of primary alcohols (apart from ethanol), aldehydes, ketones and esters, as well as various salts and acids. Some are derived from grains, grapes or other vegetable sources; some develop during fermentation. Others enter during ageing

Table XII. Chemical constituents of beers [1,2]

Component	Unit	Range	Lager	Malt liquor	Ale	Bock	Stout	Danish	Dutch	German
Carbon dioxide	%	0.45–0.55	0.51	0.50	0.51	0.49	0.50	0.50	0.52	0.49
Fluoride	ppm	0.1–0.9	0.5		0.1					
Hydrogen sulphide	ppm	Tr–0.10	0.01	0.02	0.03			0.02	0.01	0.02
Phosphate	ppm	50–350	150							
Sulphur dioxide	ppm	1–20	4.9	5.4	5		6.0	4.8	4.0	5.0
Calcium	ppm	20–70	40		64	60				
Copper	ppm	Tr–0.40	0.16	0.18	0.15			0.10	0.07	0.17
Iron	ppm	Tr–0.64	0.10	0.15	0.16			0.07	0.13	0.19
Magnesium	ppm	50–300	200			52				
Potassium	ppm	130–1040	400			420				427
Sodium	ppm	68–550	70							
Methyl alcohol	ppm	0								
Ethyl alcohol	% (vol)	2.9–7.5	4.84	6.41	4.73	5.73	6.97	5.10	4.75	5.61
Ethyl alcohol	% (wt)	2.3–6.0	3.87	5.14	3.79	4.59	5.60	4.08	3.80	4.49
Higher alcohols	ppm	42–76	60							
Diacetyl	ppm	0.03–1.00	0.12	0.20	0.16			0.10	0.08	0.09
Acetaldehyde	ppm	2.3–19.5	9.1							
pH		3.90–4.70	4.34	4.41	4.42	4.32	4.00	4.32	4.35	4.52
Lactic acid	%	0.08–0.50	0.13	0.15	0.11	0.21	0.48	0.14	0.15	0.17
Total carbohydrate	%	2.1–8.3	5.0		4.15	3.42				
Hexoses	%		1.25	1.26	1.52	1.92	1.13	1.22	1.12	1.35
Total esters	ppm	23–55	40							
Tannins	ppm	100–385	211	199	192			185	270	295

Isohumulones	ppm	6–40	22	11	20			25	27	30
Protein	ppm	630–6160	3160	3700	3350	5700	5200	2650	2850	3930
Amino acids	ppm		210							
Ammonia	ppm	5–40								
Thiamine	µg/litre	20–60	50							42
Riboflavin	µg/litre	300–1200	500			250				249
Pantothenic acid	µg/litre	400–900	500			550				
Pyridoxine	µg/litre	400–900	600			592	770			470
Nicotinic acid	µg/litre	5,000–20,000	10,000			6340				8500
Biotin	µg/litre	0–15	5							
Total solids	%	2.79–6.10	4.53	3.87	4.80	6.04	4.98	4.09	4.06	4.59

1 Average values given.
2 From Leake and Silverman (1971).

and storage (such as tannin which enters bourbon from specially charred casks). Some are deliberately added to vary the colour or flavour. For example, whisky is often coloured with caramel and may be treated with small amounts of sherry, prune juice, honey, glycerol, oak-chip extracts, fruit extracts, sugar and other ingredients. It is of interest that in addition to many of the compounds found in other beverages, beer also contains considerable amounts of carbohydrate and some peptides and other protein derivatives. These can account for up to half the caloric value of some beers.

The possible significance of congeners in producing physiological and pathological changes has been the subject of many reviews (Leake and Silverman, 1971; Murphree, 1971; see also suppl. 5 of Quarterly Journal of Studies on Alcohol, 1970). At first glance, one might be tempted to predict that because of its very much higher concentration, ethanol would produce toxic changes long before any effects of other compounds would become apparent. However, many of the congeners, notably furfural, have an LD_{50} in rats that is 10 to 100 times higher than that for ethanol (Haag et al., 1959). Thus even low concentrations could be significant. However, progress in this field has been painstakingly slow. The minute amounts of the different congeners and their volatility has presented major methodological problems. Earlier studies used distillation techniques and chemical methods to distinguish such groups as total acids, esters, aldehydes, furfural, tannins and fusel oil. The latter is an oily liquid with a disagreeable taste that remains after distilling off the ethanol. It contains most of the congeners. The advent of gas-liquid chromatography has allowed the separation of literally dozens of chemical constituents. The problem is compounded by the endless variability in congener content of alcoholic drinks. This applies especially to wines in which some variation will be demonstrable even from one bin to the next (as would be expected, considering the differences in taste and aroma).

Because of these problems, one approach has been to compare the effects of two alcoholic beverages of known high and low congener content but of equal ethanol content. A common comparison is that of vodka with bourbon. These have the lowest and highest congener contents respectively of common spirits, i.e. 3.3mg per 100ml and 285.6mg per 100ml (Carroll, 1970). Murphree (1971) reviewed a number of such studies in animals, fish and humans, which showed significant differences in physiological and behavioural reactivity between the effects of these two beverages. The studies included objective changes such as the development of nystagmus and abnormal EEG responses. These results together with observed changes in ethanol absorption with different beverages (see section 2.2.3), leave little doubt that the congeners can contribute to the overall effects of alcoholic beverages. However, in the opinion of the author, it remains to be shown that these effects are of practical importance and not just of academic interest.

Table XIII. Chemical constituents of table wines[1]

Components	Unit	Range	Red	Rosé	Dry White	Sweet White	Champagne
Carbon dioxide	%	0.01–0.05[2]					1.5
Chloride[3]	ppm	10–80	35	40	33	30	30
Sulphate	ppm	70–1000	680	600	700	700	600
Sulphur dioxide	ppm	0–590	109	120	142	171	88
Calcium	ppm	29–99	62	70	63	61	67
Copper	ppm	0–9	0.2	0.1	0.2	0.2	0.3
Iron	ppm	0–20	6.0	3.0	4.7	3.8	7.5
Potassium	ppm	180–1620	794	673	780	698	740
Sodium[4]	ppm	10–200	85	160	113	97	68
Methyl alcohol	ppm	20–230					
Ethyl alcohol	%(vol)	10.2–14.2	12.2	12.2	11.9	12.4	12.5
Higher alcohols	ppm	140–417	298	249	254	218	246
Glycerol	%	0.4–1.5	0.9	0.8	0.7	0.9	0.7
Acetaldehyde	ppm	5–292	46	80	91	128	83
pH		2.84–4.07	3.68	3.45	3.52	3.50	3.20
Acetic acid	ppm	220–1490	470	290	290	430	500
Citric acid	ppm	Tr–500					
Lactic acid	%	0.1–0.5	0.2		0.2		
Succinic acid	ppm	500–2000					
Tartaric acid	%	0.4–1.1	0.6	0.6	0.6	0.6	0.7
Hexoses[5]	%	0.02–4.80	0.21	1.12	0.29	4.07	1.50
Pentoses	%	0.08–0.20					
Total esters	ppm	60–557	280	260	244	288	191
Volatile esters	ppm	19–192	79	73	68	80	34
Tannins	%	0.01–0.36	0.18	0.05	0.03	0.03	0.04
Amino acids	ppm	100–2000					
Choline	ppm	17–41					
Mesoinositol	ppm	220–730					
Thiamine	µg/litre	0–240	10	10	20		
Riboflavin	µg/litre	60–220	130	130	90		
Pantothenic acid	µg/litre	70–450	370	290	370		
Pyridoxine	µg/litre	220–820	470	370	260		
Nicotinic acid	µg/litre		960	410	570		
Cyanocobalamin	mµg/litre	9–25	12	10	3		
Folic acid	µg/litre		15	21	18		
Biotin	µg/litre	0.6–4.6					
Total solids[6]	%	1.7–8.3	2.9	2.6	2.4	5.7	3.3

1 Average values given for specific wines. From Leake and Silverman (1971)
2 Range values of 0.01–0.05% apply only to normal still (nonsparkling) wines
3 Higher values have been reported from wines produced in European coastal areas
4 Values indicated here apply to most wines. Higher values, up to 815ppm, have been found in some American and European wines treated with ion exchange resins.
5 Usually the hexoses occur as glucose and fructose in a l : l ratio. In certain products, such as so-called kosher wines, the beverages are artificially sweetened, and the sugar content may be as high as 15% or more.
6 Customarily the total solids of wines are described as 'total extract'.

Table XIV. Congener content of spirits (g per 100 litres at 50% alcohol)[1]

Beverage	1[2]	2	3	4	5	6	7	Totals
Smirnoff vodka	0.44	0.50	0	0.49	0	1.35	0.52	3.30
Gordon's gin	0.33	0.40	0.06	2.33	0.06	1.17	0	4.35
Seagram's VO whisky	1.71	1.11	14.70	2.82	2.19	5.56	18.45	46.54
Bacardi Silver L. rum	4.18	1.88	13.75	1.44	10.62	4.56	23.70	60.13
Cutty Sark whisky	3.14	1.55	32.71	3.49	14.90	24.40	30.25	110.44
Seagram 7 crown whisky	1.69	0.96	40.70	1.98	4.54	18.60	62.10	130.57
Hennessy cognac	7.14	3.93	53.58	14.76	16.67	39.60	116.60	252.28
Old Crow whisky	1.98	3.14	96.00	3.04	12.80	29.10	139.50	285.56
Synthetic alcohol	0.16	0.42	0	0.46	0	0	0	1.04
Grain neutral spirits	0.09	0.95	0.08	0.48	1.63	0	0	3.23

1 From Carroll, 1970.
2 1, acetaldehyde; 2, ethyl formate; 3, ethyl acetate; 4, methanol; 5, n-propanol; 6, i-butanol; 7, i-amyl alcohol.

Generally speaking, the neuropharmacologic effects of the congeners are qualitatively similar (Murphree, 1971). The main differences are only in regard to potency and duration of action. Most congeners produce gastrointestinal irritation when taken orally followed by an intoxication similar to that produced by ethanol and the volatile anaesthetics. There is dizziness, light-headedness, and excitement followed by lassitude and drowsiness. Large doses produce nausea, vomiting, headache, respiratory depression and death in coma.

The neuropharmacologic effects of the congeners appear to be partly additive to those of ethanol. It is tempting to attribute them mainly to the higher alcohols, especially n-propanol, isobutanol and isoamyl alcohol since these are present in the largest amounts. However, their duration of action, when taken with ethanol, appears to be longer than might be expected from their rates of metabolism (Murphree, 1971). The explanation may be a competitive inhibition in the ADH pathway. The higher alcohols are predominantly metabolized by this pathway, but also by the microsomal alcohol oxidizing system, and their metabolism is inhibited in the presence of ethanol (Aebi and von Wartburg, 1960; Greenberg, 1970).

Apart from the acute toxic effects, the congeners have also been implicated in the production of 'hangovers' and delirium tremens (see Kissin, 1974b). Studies of the 'hangover' effect have generally shown a greater effect with bourbon than with vodka, but these investigations have been poorly controlled and no firm conclusions can be drawn from them. Other studies have suggested a possible role for methanol, acetaldehyde and formaldehyde in delirium tremens. A hypertensive crisis is sometimes seen in patients receiving MAO inhibitors and drinking wine or beer. The high tyramine content of these beverages is largely responsible (see section 7.4.1). A dramatic outbreak of 'alcoholic cardiomyopathy' in Quebec was eventually found to be due to a change in production methods by a local brewery (Morin and Daniel, 1967). The addition of cobalt to beer to steady the 'head' or foam had been introduced in the 1960's and a number of other cases were soon discovered in other parts of the world. There is indirect evidence to suggest that alcoholism could in some way 'sensitize' the heart to the toxic effects of heavy metals such as cobalt and arsenic (Morin and Daniel, 1967). One could speculate that drinking alcohol could also alter the responses of the myocardium to other drugs, thus producing a direct interaction secondary to metabolic changes in the target organ.

9. Miscellaneous Experimental Aspects

9.1 Alcohol Diets

Most animals have a natural aversion to alcohol. Wallgren and Barry (1970) have exhaustively reviewed the factors influencing the voluntary intake of alcohol by animals. These include such diverse influences as the concentration of ethanol, the presence or absence of other additives, the size, shape and position of feeding bottles, the associated dietary intake, temperature, light, time of day and genetic factors. In the majority of studies, ethanol was given as an addition to the drinking water of the animals. However, despite the enormous number of studies using this method of alcohol administration the spontaneous intake is commonly so low as to result in undetectable blood ethanol levels. Various authors have tried the addition of sucrose to the ethanol solutions but evidence that this significantly enhances ethanol intake has not been consistently produced. Ethanol blood levels in fish are easily controlled by varying the ethanol concentration of the fluid in which they swim. However, the results of such studies are even more difficult to extrapolate to human investigations than those carried out in more conventional laboratory species. An analogous technique in animals is the administration of ethanol by inhalation. This has been given in a sealed chamber to rats receiving pyrazole, an inhibitor of ADH, to maintain high blood levels (Goldstein and Nandita, 1971). However the equipment required for this is cumbersome, and pyrazole itself is hepatotoxic (Lieber et al., 1970). Various other techniques that have been tried to achieve reasonable blood alcohol levels in animals have included:

1) chronic intravenous administration in monkeys, either externally programmed or self-administered through operant responding

2) intraperitoneal injections

3) repeated intragastric inhalation

4) instillation through an intragastric cannula.

Intraperitoneal injections give a very rapid rise in blood ethanol but should be avoided because of the toxicity of high local concentrations bathing the abdominal organs. This can produce chemical peritonitis and hepatic necrosis (Strubelt et al., 1972). Drawbacks common to all these methods include their complexity and the marked reduction in appetite which is produced. A variable and uncontrolled intake of food makes it impossible to distinguish between the effects directly due to ethanol and those due to an altered intake of other compounds of the diet.

A dietary regimen that overcomes these objections is that introduced by De Carli and Lieber (1967). Ethanol (providing 36 per cent of total calories) is incorporated in a totally liquid diet in a concentration of 5g per 100ml (table XV). This is given in calibrated Richter tubes to animals housed in individual cages. A convenient, slightly modified preparation can now be obtained commercially (Bio-Serv Inc., Little Silver, N.J.). The technique has the following advantages:

a) ethanol is taken orally and spontaneously; forced feeding is avoided;

b) ethanol intake is of the order of 15—16g/kg/day, that is, approximately double that achieved by adding ethanol to drinking water and even higher than that obtained by rats inbred for their preference for ethanol (Eriksson, 1972);

c) the technique of pair-feeding is greatly facilitated;

d) all nutritional components are defined and the control animals can be fed with equal amounts of a diet identical in composition except for the isocaloric replacement of ethanol by carbohydrate;

e) the diet can be fairly readily modified to allow variations in practically any of the dietary constituents. For example, ethanol can be isocalorically replaced by fat instead of carbohydrate. This could be important where it is thought that the differences between the test animals and their controls might be due to differences in carbohydrate rather than to ethanol intake (Baraona et al., 1974).

With this method there is a tendency for the restricted control rats to drink their daily supply shortly after feeding, while the 'alcohol rats' maintain a relatively steady intake throughout the day. Thus in some experiments it is necessary to feed at frequent intervals, especially in the last day before testing. This liquid diet has been widely used in studies of the role of ethanol in the

Table XV. Composition of control liquid diet (Lieber and De Carli, 1970d)

Substance	Per litre
Micropulverized casein	41.4g
L-Cystine	0.5g
DL-Methionine	0.3g
Vitamin Mixture[1]	5.0g
'Hegsted' salt mixture	10.0g
Corn oil	8.5g
Olive oil	28.5g
Ethyl linoleate	2.7g
Vitamin A acetate	2.0mg
Calciferol	0.01mg
DL-α-tocopherol acetate	30.0mg
Dextrin-maltose	115.9g[2]
Sodium carragheenate[3]	2.5g
Distilled water	to 1 litre

1 Contains, in milligrams, thiamin, 0.725; riboflavin, 1.25; pyridoxine hydrochloride, 0.725; calcium pantothenate, 5.0; nicotinamide, 3.75; choline chloride, 250.0; biotin, 0.025; folic acid, 0.25; inositol, 25.0; 2 methyl-1,4 naphthoquinone, 0.25; vitamin B_{12}, 0.025; p-aminobenzoic acid, 12.5; and glucose, 4,700.50.
2 Replaced by 24.9g dextrin-maltose and 50.0g ethanol in the ethanol formula.
3 Purchased as Viscarin TP-4 from Marine Colloids, Inc., Springfield, New Jersey.

production of alcoholic fatty liver and alcoholic hyperlipaemia in the rat (Lieber, 1973a) and provides an alcohol intake sufficient to produce withdrawal seizures on cessation of ethanol (Lieber and De Carli, 1973b). However, neither this, nor other previous methods of alcohol feeding resulted in alcoholic hepatitis or cirrhosis in laboratory animals. This was presumably because even with this method of alcohol feeding, the high alcohol intake of humans could not be matched. Using a modification of this liquid diet for the feeding of baboons, Lieber and De Carli (1974) were able to supply 50 per cent of total calories in the form of ethanol. This regimen led to the appearance of alcoholic hepatitis and alcoholic cirrhosis in these animals (Rubin and Lieber, 1974). This appears to be an important advance in the development of animal models in alcoholism.

9.2 'Acute' and 'Chronic' Alcohol Intake

At first sight, the distinction between the acute and the chronic intake of ethanol seems easy. By convention, an acute effect is that produced shortly after a single dose and a chronic effect is that produced by repeated intake over at least a few days. However, a number of problems can arise if careful attention is not paid to the time of feeding. For example, some studies of the effects of ethanol on hepatic drug-metabolizing enzymes and on intestinal function have been carried out 16 hours after a single dose of ethanol. This lapse of time may be sufficient to allow some of the 'inducing' effects of ethanol on the hepatic SER to start to appear. Similarly, in 16 hours there may be a secondary rise in intestinal villous enzyme activity quite distinct from the suppression that occurs within the first hour (Baraona et al., 1974).

The assessment of chronic alcohol intake can be even more difficult. The continued intake of ethanol even up to the time of testing will not allow a clear distinction to be made between its acute and chronic effects because some ethanol will still be present. At least this has the advantage that it tends to mimic the clinical situation of the alcoholic who is commonly responding to both the acute and the chronic intake of ethanol. Furthermore, the chronic effects may be merely an exaggeration of the acute effects. However, if they are opposing (as in the example of the villous enzymes quoted above), then misleading results may be obtained. Of course a prolonged fast will ensure the full elimination of ethanol from the body, but fasting itself may obscure an important metabolic effect of ethanol such as an enhanced capacity for hepatic lipoprotein output (Baraona et al., 1973). In that case, it may be necessary to feed an isocaloric control diet in the 12–14 hours before testing. Another problem associated with the cessation of ethanol is the possible development of subclinical features of delirium tremens so that the 'chronic' effect of alcohol becomes obscured by the acute features of withdrawal.

9.3 Congeners

The studies of the effects of congeners is fraught with problems (see section 8). These are mainly due to the very small and unpredictable concentrations of the congeners in most drinks, and their volatility. Therefore a standard approach is to design an experiment that tests the effects of the total congener content. The underlying assumption is that if no effect is demonstrable, then a more detailed study of individual congeners may not be warranted. An extension of this approach is to isolate the total congeners of a beverage and to administer these to animals. Alternatively one can concentrate the congener content of a beverage such as bourbon (known for its high concentration of these substances) and thus produce a 'super bourbon' for testing (Murphree et al., 1967). A simpler approach is to compare a beverage of known high congener content such as bourbon with a solution of ethanol or with a beverage of known low congener content such as vodka (see section 8). For chronic congener studies of this type, the liquid diet of De Carli and Lieber (1967) can be used. The constituents of the diet (with appropriate reductions in water and ethanol) are added to the beverage being studied. Pair feeding is then carried out with animals receiving the congener-free ethanol diet. However this normally has an alcohol concentration of 5g per 100ml, so that suitable congener diets cannot normally be made up from beverages with an alcohol content of less than this value. This applies to most North American and European beers.

9.4 Intravenous Administration and Blood Alcohol Levels

The intravenous administration of ethanol has the advantage of providing a rapid and predictable blood alcohol level. It also avoids the direct stimulation (or inhibition) of the alimentary tract by high local concentrations of alcohol. However, an effect mediated through the alimentary tract (e.g. stimulation of gastrin secretion) cannot be completely excluded even by intravenous injection, because of the rapid distribution of ethanol in body fluids. Another advantage of the intravenous route is avoidance of excessively high concentrations of ethanol in the portal circulation (and therefore presumably in the liver) such as occurs after oral ingestion (Beck et al., 1974). Disadvantages include the inconvenience and usual hazards of intravenous injections and the difficulty of providing a suitable control (particularly with respect to the osmolality of the injected fluid). A loading dose of approximately 600mg per kg followed by a constant infusion of 3mg per kg will tend to maintain a constant blood level of about 50–60mg per 100ml. The relationship of dose to blood levels and the factors influencing the shape of the blood alcohol curve are discussed in detail by Loomis (1950) and Kalant (1971) respectively. It should be noted that the levels of alcohol in the blood fluctuate erratically and unpredictably during and for several minutes after a rapid infusion of ethanol. Presumably these changes are due to rapid changes in tissue distribution. Once the peak is reached after a single infusion, the rate of fall is remarkably constant (approximately 15 to 20mg per 100ml per hour) until a level below 9mg/100ml (2mM) is reached. The rapid distribution of ethanol in body fluids is fortuitous because it allows estimations of the tissue levels of ethanol to be made simply by measuring its concentration in the blood. This contrasts with other drug studies which are complicated by such factors as plasma protein binding and cell uptake. The flattening of the blood alcohol curve at low concentrations presumably reflects lack of saturation of ADH. Some authors have reported that the rest of the descending limb is linear at all blood concentrations of ethanol; others have claimed that the curve is steeper at high concentrations (see Wallgren and Barry, 1970).

It is important to bear in mind the K_ms for ADH and for MEOS (2 and 8.6mM respectively) when designing a study involving either of these two enzyme systems. For example if it is designed to test a hypothesis related to the activity of ADH then a blood concentration of over 25mg per 100ml will be adequate to achieve saturation of ADH. Higher doses will not significantly affect ADH activity but will introduce all sorts of variables due to the other physiological and pathological effects of ethanol. For example, if an alcoholic is found to have a more severe degree of lactic acidosis when the blood alcohol level is 150mg per 100ml than when it is 100mg per 100ml, then it would be most unwise to ascribe the difference to altered lactate production secondary to the effects of ADH (see section 5.1.4). At both blood levels of alcohol, ADH should be fully saturated and other factors such as hypoxia should be sought to explain the findings. Similarly, if an effect based on MEOS activity is being investigated, it is desirable to maintain blood levels above 80mg per 100ml.

9.5 Radio-isotope Studies of Ethanol Metabolism

Radio-isotope studies have proved useful in the assessment of total body metabolism of ethanol. ^{14}C-ethanol is given with a dose of unlabelled ethanol sufficient to give a blood alcohol level appropriate to the aims of the study. The rate of excretion of ^{14}CO$_2$ in the expired air is then recorded.

Similar methods have been applied to the study of the relative rates of ethanol metabolism in different organs. These experiments give information concerning the conversion of ethanol to CO_2 by different organs but this is a misleading indication of ethanol metabolism *in vivo*. The underlying assumption is that each organ normally converts most of the ethanol to CO_2. This is certainly not the case with the liver, where the major product of ethanol oxidation is acetate which is then converted to CO_2 by other tissues (see section 5.6). Direct conversion of ethanol to CO_2 in the liver is negligible. Thus it is not surprising that comparisons of other organs using the above method have yielded comparable and even higher rates of ^{14}CO$_2$ production from ^{14}C-ethanol than those obtained with the liver. These studies have included comparisons of rat hepatic and renal slices (Bartlett and Barnett, 1949), perfused canine liver and perfused hind limb of the dog, which is 50 per cent muscle (Forsander and Räihä, 1960), and rat hepatic, gastric and small intestinal slices (Carter and Isselbacher, 1971b). The last-mentioned study exemplifies the problems associated with this method. From the authors' data it can be calculated that under the conditions of the study, rat hepatic slices converted ethanol to CO_2 at a rate of 15.5 x 10^{-9} gm of ethanol per gm of tissue per hour. If this were representative of ethanol metabolism *in vivo*, then it would take the average person months to eliminate the alcohol from a bottle of beer.

9.6 Microsomal Enzyme Induction

Studies of microsomal enzyme induction require considerable attention to detail if complicating and uncontrolled influences are to be avoided. Examples of unwanted complications that may occur are given in section 4.5. The paired feeding of littermates eliminates a number of nutritional and hereditary variables. Controlled temperature, light and the general cleanliness of animal quarters are vital. Insecticides that contain halogenated hydrocarbons should be avoided, but Pyrethrum has not been shown to stimulate drug metabolism.

9.6.1 Tests of Enzyme Induction

Direct proof of enzyme induction requires evidence that the administration of an inducing agent produces an increase in the specific activity of the enzyme in question. Assays suitable for needle biopsies have been used in human studies (Schoene et al., 1972). The range of enzymes induced by most inducing agents is surprisingly wide (see section 4.4.1). However, evidence that microsomal enzyme induction has taken place cannot be taken as evidence that the metabolism of a specific drug will be enhanced, since the spectrum of enzymes induced and the magnitude of the changes will vary according to the inducing agent (Conney, 1971). The analysis of cytochrome P-450 can be useful because its concentration generally increases in proportion to the extent of the enzyme induction. However, there are exceptions. For example, the hepatic microsomal concentration of cytochrome P-450 is increased by phenobarbital and 3-methylcholanthrene but only the former enhances the metabolism of benzphetamine and aniline (Peters, 1973), and there are differences in the type of cytochrome P-450 that is induced (Levin and Kuntzman, 1969; Comai and Gaylor, 1973).

Indirect indications of enzyme induction are commonly obtained from *in vivo* studies by measuring the half-life of a drug or by showing an increased rate of appearance of a metabolite in the blood or urine. Hexobarbital and zoxazolamine are two drugs commonly used for clearance studies. The simplest method is to measure the duration of action of these drugs. For example rats can be injected intraperitoneally twice daily with hexobarbital 100mg/kg for four days. On the fifth day a test dose of 120mg/kg can be given and the sleeping time recorded. Theoretically, changes in pharmacodynamic tolerance can complicate the enhanced metabolic tolerance so that measurements of plasma levels provide more precise information concerning the presence or absence of enzyme induction. The use of both hexobarbital and zoxazolamine in such studies is valuable because the relative clearance of these drugs gives an indication of the type of microsomal change that is occurring. For example, nonspecific inducers such as phenobarbital enhance the metabolism of both drugs, whereas only zoxazolamine metabolism is increased by 3-methylcholanthrene. Other drugs commonly used in plasma clearance studies of enzyme induction are pentobarbital, aminopyrine, antipyrine (which has the advantage of being evenly distributed in body water) and phenylbutazone.

The measurement of urinary metabolites has also been used, especially in human experiments. The urinary levels of D-glucaric acid and ascorbic acid have been found to be helpful in a number of investigations. Microsomal enzyme induction enhances the metabolism of glucose and galactose via the glucuronic acid pathway through D-glucuronic acid and L-gulonic acid. This results in an increased synthesis of glucaric acid and ascorbic acid. Changes in urinary steroid levels have also been used. Inducing agents commonly enhance the β-hydroxylation of steroids. Thus the ratio of urinary 6β-hydroxycortisol to total urinary 17-hydrocorticosteroids is raised.

The plasma level of some hepatic enzymes is increased following chronic drug administration. This applies especially to γ-glutamyl transpeptidase (GGT) whose activity is raised in patients on anticonvulsant therapy and in heavy drinkers. This observation led to the hope that the enzyme might serve as a simple indicator of enzyme induction. Whitfield et al. (1973) studied the relationship between rises in the plasma levels of GGT and stimulation of warfarin metabolism by various drugs. There was some correlation between the two, but their conclusion was that plasma GGT activity could not always be used as an index of hepatic drug metabolism since a number of both false-positive and false-negative results was obtained.

Another indirect indication of enhanced microsomal enzyme activity is the demonstration of proliferation of the endoplasmic reticulum. A common method of assessment of this is by electron microscopy (Fouts and Rogers, 1965). A marked prominence of the hepatic SER is characteristic of animals treated with phenobarbital, tolbutamide, DDT and other agents. Drugs with a narrower range of inducing activity such as 3-methylcholanthrene, produce less obvious changes in the SER. Ethanol-induced proliferation of the hepatic SER is well documented. However, quantitation of these morphological changes is difficult. A more reliable indication of increased microsomal mass is measurement of its major constituents, namely phospholipid and protein (see section 5.4.3).

9.6.2 Choice of Inducing Agents

Remmer (1969, 1972) has summarised the properties required of a chemical substance for it to be capable of enzyme induction:

1) It should be lipid soluble. Generally speaking, the greater the ratio of lipid-solubility to water-solubility, the greater is the capacity for induction. Exceptions are most of the alkaloids such as pethidine and morphine, which are not inducing agents.

2) The drug should behave as a type I compound by binding to the protein moiety of cytochrome P-450.

3) The duration of the reaction with the enzyme is important. Thus phenobarbital (despite its lower lipid solubility) is a much more potent inducer than hexobarbital because its half-life is about 11 times longer. The short-acting barbiturates are highly lipid-soluble and bind strongly to the enzyme but have a

very poor inducing capacity because they are rapidly oxidized and detached from the enzyme.

4) The inducing agent must either be present in the liver in high concentration or must have a high affinity for the enzyme. Many drugs such as anticoagulants and pethidine kill the animal before they can reach a sufficiently high concentration in the liver.

In choosing an inducing agent, one should also bear in mind that testing for induction with another drug may not be possible if the inducing agent is still present. This will be especially likely to occur if the test agent has a low binding affinity for cytochrome P-450. Thus when a standard four-day inducing course of phenobarbital (80mg per kg per day) is given to rats, detectable levels of phenobarbital are still present 24 hours after the last injection. This could interfere with tests of enzyme induction since these are traditionally carried out on the fifth day. Indeed, this has been shown to be the case with the assessment of the microsomal oxidation of ethanol. This problem can be overcome by delaying the test of microsomal enzyme activity by a further day or by using hexobarbital as an inducing agent.

The pharmacological properties of an inducing agent can be an important consideration. This applies especially to therapeutic uses and to some experimental studies. Ideally, the inducing drug should be pharmacologically inactive. From this point of view, phenobarbital with its hypnotic and addicting properties, is at a disadvantage. Phetharbital and d-mephobarbital are barbiturates said to be free of hypnotic effects. Because of this, phetharbital has been tried in the treatment of neonatal jaundice. However, in rats, some degree of neuropharmacologic activity can be demonstrated with these agents (unpublished observations).

The relative potency of inducing agents in humans has not been extensively studied. Phenobarbital has been the mainstay of most investigators. Latham et al. (1973) compared four anticonvulsant drugs using urinary D-glucaric acid excretion as an indicator of induction. Pheneturide was found to have the greatest effect, followed by primidone and then phenytoin and phenobarbitone (which appeared to be of about equal potency). It would be interesting to compare these agents by other more direct tests of enzyme induction.

9.7 Alcohol-Drug Interactions

The classification of drug interactions as direct and indirect (see section 1.4) emphasises the importance of plasma levels in elucidating the mechanisms of abnormal drug responses. The most obvious drug interactions are usually direct ones involving the primary pharmacological actions of the drugs in question. Ethanol is mainly a central nervous system depressant. Thus its more important drug interactions involve other neuropharmacologically active agents. Sedatives such as the barbiturates tend to enhance its effects and stimulants tend to reduce them. The methodological problems involved in studying direct alcohol-drug interactions in humans have been summarised by Landauer and Milner (1971). These are particularly applicable to interactions involving driving safety:

1) Because of the abnormal experimental circumstances, the subject may make a great effort to perform well. The degree of concentration during the carrying out of psychomotor tasks, such as in a simulated driving test, contrast with the relative inattention devoted to such routine activities in daily life. Thus the absence of a demonstrable drug interaction in an experimental situation does not include the possibility that it exists to a significant extent under less controlled circumstances such as when the subject is bored, tired or preoccupied. Conversely, an effect observed in a laboratory may manifest itself more strongly in other circumstances.

2) The small size of treatment groups in most experiments is such that uncommon drug interactions (such as might occur in less than 5 per cent of the population) may be missed, especially when considering the average results of a group. Yet such reactions could involve an appreciable percentage of vehicle accidents and their detection could be a matter of considerable concern to the community.

3) There is a tendency for experimental subjects to consist mainly of young adults. This homogeneity has advantages in reducing the variability of responses. It could be a disadvantage if the slower reaction times of older subjects are of more practical relevance to the drug interaction being studied.

4) The state of health of the subject can be important. For example desipramine tends to act as a stimulant in depressed patients but as a sedative in healthy volunteers. Its onset of action is slower in health than in depression. By contrast, imipramine has a faster onset of action in patients than in healthy controls.

5) The effect of practice has to be taken into account. Even the well-known lengthening of the reaction time by ethanol can be reduced by practice.

6) Because of the variable factors controlling the disposal of a drug, the achievement of an adequate plasma concentration of a drug is crucial and the dosage may have to be reviewed in the light of plasma levels.

7) The time course of action in the drug should be considered. The timing of the tests and questionnaires is important. In this regard it is interesting to note the different responses to the same plasma level of ethanol, according to whether the subject is on the ascending or descending limb of the blood alcohol curve.

8) The congener contents of alcoholic beverages may affect the responses, either by a direct pharmacological action, or by interfering with ethanol absorption or metabolism. For this reason it is often preferable to give alcohol as a pure solution of ethanol in water.

9) When considering the role of drugs in road accidents, ideally every drug should be tested for its effects on judgement, mood, perception and psychomotor skills related to driving ability. Several doses, involving acute and chronic studies, should be used. The numbers should be as large as possible and should involve healthy as well as sick subjects. Major surveys, with efficient screening, are needed to compare the patterns of drug use in those involved in accidents with those in suitable controls.

Indirect drug-alcohol reactions are also important, but may be less obvious. The major factors that may be involved include changes in absorption, distribution, metabolism and excretion. A number of other influences may be present and can be easily overlooked. Some of the difficulties in studying inherited variations in drug responses are discussed in sections 4.3 and 4.3.1. Dayton and Perel (1972) have drawn attention to the following variables in studies of drug interactions:

1) The physicochemical properties of the drugs involved.

2) Species differences, e.g. protein binding in humans is generally higher than in animals.

3) Individual differences in humans.

4) Several interactions may take place simultaneously or sequentially between two drugs.

5) Physiological factors can interact with and modify physicochemical factors.

6) Metabolites may cause interactions that differ from those of the parent substances.

7) Deuterium-tagged isotopes may have different pharmacological and physicochemical characteristics that differ from the natural substances.

References

Abeles, R.H. and Lee, H.A.: The dismutation of formaldehyde by liver alcohol dehydro-genase. J. Biol. Chem. 235: 1499–1503 (1960).

Aebi, H. and von Wartburg, J.-P.: Vergleichend-biologische Aspekte der experimentellen Erforschung Chronischer Alkoholwirkungen. Bull. Schweiz. Akad. Med. Wiss. 16: 25–35 (1960).

Akabane, J.; Nakanishi, S.; Kohei, H.; Matsumura, R. and Ogata, H.: Studies on sympatho-mimetic action of acetaldehyde. I. Experiments with blood pressure and nictitating membrane responses. Japan J. Pharmacol. 14: 295–307 (1964).

A.M.A. Gazette: High School drunkness in U.S. 'amazes'. Sydney, August 8, 1974.

Amerine, M.A.: The search for good wine. Science 154: 1621–1628 (1966).

Andersen, K.L.; Hellstrom, B. and Lorentzen, F.V.: Combined effect of cold and alcohol on heat balance in man. J. App. Physiol. 18: 975–982 (1963).

Anton, A.H.: Ethanol and urinary catecholamines in man. Clin. Pharmacol. Therap. 6: 462–469 (1965).

Ariyoshi, T.; Takabatake, E. and Remmer, H.: Drug metabolism in ethanol induced fatty liver. Life Sci. 9: 361–369 (1970).

Arky, R.A.: The effect of alcohol on carbohydrate metabolism: carbohydrate metabolism in alcoholics; Ch. 6, in Kissin and Begleiter, The Biology of Alcoholism, vol. 1: Biochemistry (Plenum Press, New York 1971).

Arky, R.A.; Veverbrants, E. and Abramson, E.A.: Irreversible hypoglycemia. A complica-tion of alcohol and insulin. J. Am. Med. Ass. 206: 575–578 (1968).

Asmussen, E.; Hald, J. and Larsen, V.: The pharmacological action of acetaldehyde on the human organism. Acta Pharmacol. 4: 311–320 (1948).

Atwater, W.O. and Benedict, F.G.: An experimental inquiry regarding the nutritive value of alcohol. Mem. Nat. Acad. Science 8: 231–288 (1896).

Axelrod, J.; Inscoe, J.K. and Daly, J.: Enzymatic formation of O-methylated dihydroxy derivates from phenolic amines and indoles. J. Pharmacol. Exper. Ther. 149: 16—22 (1965).

Banks, W.L.; Kline, E.S. and Higgins, E.S.: Hepatic composition and metabolism after ethanol consumption in rats fed liquid purified diets. J. Nutr. 100: 581—594 (1970).

Baraona, E.; Pirola, R.C. and Lieber, C.S.: The pathogenesis of post-prandial hyperlipemia in rats fed ethanol-containing diets. J. Clin. Invest. 52: 296—303 (1973).

Baraona, E.; Pirola, R.C. and Lieber, C.S.: Small intestinal damage and changes in cell population produced by ethanol ingestion in the rat. Gastroenterology 66: 226—234 (1974).

Barboriak, J.J. and Meade, R.C.: Effect of alcohol on gastric emptying in man. Am. J. Clin. Nutr. 23: 1151—1153 (1970).

Barnes, E.W.; Cooke, N.J.; King, A.J. and Passmore, R.: Observations on the metabolism of alcohol in man. Brit. J. Nutr. 19: 485—489 (1965).

Baron, P. and Trémolières, J.: Influence de l'éthanol administré à dose toxique sur les échanges respiratoires du rat. Nutritio et Dieta 10: 229—239 (1968).

Bartlett, G.R. and Barnet, H.N.: Some observations on alcohol metabolism with radioactive ethyl alcohol. Quart. J. Stud. Alc. 10: 381—397 (1949).

Beazell, J.M. and Ivey, A.C.: The influence of alcohol on the digestive tract. Quart. J. Stud. Alc. 1: 45—54 (1940).

Beck, I.T.; Paloschi, G.B.; Dinda, P.K. and Beck, M.: Effect of intragastric administration of alcohol on the ethanol concentrations and osmolality of pancreatic juice, bile and portal and peripheral blood. Gastroenterology 67: 484—489 (1974).

Beckett, A.H. and Triggs, E.J.: Enzyme induction in man caused by smoking. Nature 216: 587 (1967).

Beckman, H.: Dilemmas in Drug Therapy (W.G. Saunders Co., Philadelphia 1967).

Bennett, I.L.; Cary, F.H.; Mitchell, G.L. and Cooper, M.N.: Acute methyl alcohol poisoning: a review based on experiences in an outbreak of 323 cases. Medicine 23: 431—463 (1953).

Berger, H.J.: Chlorpromazine and ethanol combination: effects on respiration, random motor activity and conditioned avoidance-escape in mice. Quart. J. Stud. Alc. 30: 862—869 (1969).

Blair, A.H. and Vallee, B.L.: Some catalitic properties of human liver alcohol dehydrogenase. Biochemistry 5: 2026—2034 (1966).

Bledsoe, T.; Island, D.P.; Ney, R.L. and Liddle, G.W.: An effect of o,ρ,-DDD on the extra-adrenal metabolism of cortisol in man. J. Clin. Endocr. 24: 1303—1311 (1964).

Blomstrand, R.: Observations on the formation of ethanol in the intestinal tract of man. Life Sci. 10: 575—582 (1971).

Bloom, R.J. and Westerfield, W.W.: A new intermediate in the metabolism of ethanol. Biochemistry 5: 3204—3210 (1966).

Bode, C.H.; Goebell, H. and Stahler, M.: Anderungen der Alkoholdehydrogenase – Aktivitat in der Rattenleber durch Eiweissmangel und Aethanol. Z. Ges. Exper. Med. 152: 111—124 (1970).

Bode, C.; Stahler, E.; Kono, H. and Goebell, H.: Effects of ethanol on free coenzyne A, free carnitine and their fatty acid esters in rat liver. Biochim. Biophys. Acta 210: 448—455 (1970).

Böhmer, K.: Die Einwirkung einiger Arzneimittel auf den Verlauf der Blutalkoholkurve. Dtsch. Z. Ges. Ger. Med. 30: 205—212 (1938).

Bolt, H.M.: Rifampicin and oral contraceptives. Lancet 1: 1280—1281 (1974).

Bonnichsen, R.K. and Wassen, A.M.: Crystalline alcohol dehydrogenase from horse liver. Arch. Biochem. 18: 361–363 (1948).

Boveris, A.; Oshino, N. and Chance, B.: The cellular production of hydrogen peroxide. Biochem. J. 128: 617–630 (1972).

Brodie, B.B.; Axelrod, J.; Cooper, J.R.; Gaudette, L.; La Du, B.N.; Mitoma, C. and Udenfriend, S.: Detoxication of drugs and other foreign compounds by liver microsomes. Science 121: 603–604 (1955).

Brown, R.R.; Miller, J.A. and Miller, E.C.: The metabolism of methylated aminoazo dyes. IV. Dietary factors enhancing demethylation in vitro. J. Biol. Chem. 209: 211–222 (1954).

Bullar, F. and Wood, C.A.: Poisoning by wood alcohol; cases of death and blindness from Columbian spirits and other methylated preparations. J. Am. Med. Ass. 43: 972, 1058, 1117, 1213, 1289 (1904).

Burbridge, T.N. and Hine, C.H.: Studies in the metabolism of ethanol excretion of C_{14} labelled $CH_3 CH_2 OH$ in rat. J. Pharmacol. Exper. Therap. 103: 338–339 (1951).

Burstein, S. and Klaiber, E.L.: Phenobarbital-induced increase in 6β-hydroxycortisol excretion: clue to its significance in human urine. J. Clin. Endocr. 25: 293–296 (1965).

Byron, J. and Tephly, T.R.: Effect of 3-amino-1,2,4-triazole on the stimulation of hepatic microsomal heme synthesis and induction of hepatic microsomal oxidases produced by phenobarbital. Mol. Pharmacol. 5: 10–20 (1969).

Cabana, B.E. and Gessner, P.K.: The kinetics of chloral hydrate metabolism in mice and the effect thereon of ethanol. J. Pharmacol. Exper. Therap. 174: 260–275 (1970).

Carlsson, C. and Johannson, T.: The psychological effects of propranolol in the abstinence phase of chronic alcoholics. Brit. J. Psych. 119: 605–606 (1971).

Carpenter, T.M. and Lee, R.C.: The effect of fructose on the metabolism of ethyl alcohol in man. J. Pharmacol. Exper. Therap. 60: 286–295 (1937).

Carroll, L.F.: Analysis of alcoholic beverages by gas-liquid chromatography. Quart. J. Stud. Alc. Supp. 5: 6–19 (1970).

Carter, E.A. and Isselbacher, K.J.: The role of microsomes in the hepatic metabolism of ethanol. Ann. N.Y. Acad. Sci. 179: 282–294 (1971a).

Carter, E.A. and Isselbacher, K.J.: The metabolism of ethanol to carbon dioxide by stomach and small intestinal slices. Proc. Soc. Exp. Biol. Med. 138: 817–819 (1971b).

Carter, E.A. and Isselbacher, K.J.: Hepatic microsomal ethanol oxidation. Mechanism and physiological significance. Lab. Invest. 27: 283–286 (1972).

Carulli, N.; Manenti, F.; Gallo, M. and Salvioli, G.F.: Alcohol-drugs interaction in man: alcohol and tolbutamide. Eur. J. Clin. Invest. 1: 421–424 (1971).

Casier, H. and Delaunois, A.L.: Influence des dinitrodérivés, specialement du dinitrocrésol et du dinitrophénol, sur la résorption et l'élimination de l'alcool par l'organisme. Arch. Int. Pharmacodyn. Thérap. 69: 156–162 (1943).

Casier, H. and Merlevede, E.: On the mechanism of the disulfiram-ethanol intoxication symptoms. Arch. Int. Pharmacodyn. Thérap. 139: 165–176 (1962).

Casier, H. and Polet, H.: Influence du disulfiram (Antabus) sur le métabolisme de l'alcool éthylique marqué chez la souris. Arch. Int. Pharmacodyn. Thérap. 113: 439–496 (1958).

Casier, H.; Danechmand, L.; De Schaepdryver, A.; Hermans, W. and Piette, Y.: Blood alcohol levels and psychotropic drugs. Arz. Hel. Forschung. 16: 1505–1507 (1966).

Cederbaum, A.I.; Lieber, C.S.; Beattie, D.S. and Rubin, E.: Effect of chronic ethanol ingestion on mitochondrial permeability and the transport of reducing equivalents. Biochem. Biophys. Res. Comm. 49: 649–655 (1972).

Chappell, J.B.: Systems used for the transport of substrates into mitochondria. Brit. Med. Bull. 24: 150–157 (1968).

Chaudhury, R.R.; Chaudhury, M.R. and Lu, F.C.: Depressed diuresis caused by ethanol after a water load in rats. Can. J. Physiol. Pharmacol. 43: 901–904 (1964).

Chen, W.; Vrindten, P.A.; Dayton, P.G. and Burns, J.J.: Accelerated aminopyrine metabolism in human subjects pretreated with phenylbutazone. Life Sci. 1: 35–42 (1962).

Cherrick, G.R. and Leevy, C.M.: The effect of ethanol metabolism on levels of oxidized and reduced nicotinamide-adenine dinucleotide in liver, kidney and heart. Biochim. Biophys. Acta 109: 29–37 (1965).

Chey, W.Y.: Alcohol and gastric mucosa. Digestion 7: 239–251 (1972).

Chey, W.Y.; Kosay, S. and Lorber, S.H.: Effects of chronic administration of ethanol on gastric secretion of acid in dogs. Am. J. Dig. Dis. 17: 153–159 (1972).

Clark, W.C. and Hulpieu, H.R.: The disulfiram-like activity of animal charcoal. J. Pharmacol. Exper. Therap. 123: 74–80 (1958).

Closs, K.: Methanol poisoning and its treatment. Ind. Med. 40: 20–22 (1971).

Cohen, B.S. and Estabrook, B.W.: Microsomal electron transport reactions. Interaction of reduced triphosphopyridine nucleotide during the oxidative demethylation of aminopyrine and cytochrome b_5 reduction. Arch. Biochem. Biophys. 143: 37–45 (1971a).

Cohen, B.S. and Estabrook, R.W.: Microsomal electron transport reactions. III. Co-operative interactions between reduced diphosphopyridine nucleotide and reduced triphosphopyridine nucleotide linked reactions. Arch. Biochem. Biophys. 143: 54–65 (1971b).

Comai, K. and Gaylor, J.L.: Existence and separation of three forms of cytochrome P-450 from rat liver microsomes. J. Biol. Chem. 248: 4947–4955 (1973).

Conney, A.H.: Pharmacological implications of microsomal enzyme induction. Pharmacol. Rev. 19: 317–336 (1967).

Conney, A.H.: Environmental factors influencing drug metabolism; in La Du, Mandel and Way, Fundamentals of Drug Metabolism and Drug Disposition (Williams and Wilkins, Baltimore 1971).

Cooke, A.R.: Aspirin, ethanol and the stomach. Aust. Ann. Med. 19: 269–274 (1970).

Cooke, A.R. and Birchall, A.: Absorption of ethanol from the stomach. Gastroenterology 57: 269–272 (1969).

Cooke, A.R. and Grossman, M.I.: Comparison of stimulants of antral release of gastrin. Amer. J. Physiol. 215: 314–318 (1968).

Cooper, J.R. and Friedman, P.J.: The enzymic oxidation of chloral hydrate to trichloroacetic acid. Biochem. Pharmacol. 1: 76–82 (1958).

Cooper, S.D. and Feuer, G.: Effects of drugs or hepatotoxins on the relation between drug-metabolizing activity and phospholipids in hepatic microsomes during choline deficiency. Toxicol. App. Pharmacol. 25: 7–19 (1973).

Cooper, J.R. and Kini, M.M.: Biochemical aspects of methanol poisoning. Biochem. Pharmacol. 11: 405–416 (1962).

Cornish, H.H. and Adefuin, J.: Ethanol potentiation of halogenated aliphatic solvent toxicity. Am. Ind. Hyg. Ass. J. 9: 57–61 (1966).

Crigler, J.F. and Gold, N.I.: Effect of sodium phenobarbital on bilirubin metabolism in an infant with congenital, non-hemolytic, unconjugated hyperbilirubinemia and kernicterus. J. Clin. Invest. 48: 42–55 (1969).

Crompton, D.W.T. and Ward, P.F.V.: Production of ethanol and succinate by Moniliformis dubius (Acantocephala). Nature 215: 964–965 (1967).

Cucinell, S.A.; Conney, A.H.; Sansur, M. and Burns, J.J.: Drug interactions in man. I. Lowering effect of phenobarbital on plasma levels of bishydroxycoumarin (Dicumarol) and diphenylhydantoin (Dilantin). Clin. Pharmacol. Therap. 6: 420–429 (1965).

Cucinell, S.A.; Oddesky, L.; Weiss, M. and Dayton, P.G.: The effect of chloral hydrate on bishydroxycoumarin metabolism. J. Am. Med. Ass. 197: 366–368 (1966).

Dajani, R.M.; Danielski, J. and Orten, J.M.: The utilization of ethanol. II. The alcohol acetaldehyde dehydrogenase systems in the livers of alcohol treated rats. J. Nutr. 80: 196–204 (1963).

Dalziel, K. and Dickinson, F.M.: The activity of liver alcohol dehydrogenase with nicotinamide-adenine dinucleotide phosphate as coenzyme. Biochem. J. 95: 311–321 (1965).

Damgaard, E.; Lundquist, F.; Tonneson, K.; Hansen, F.V. and Sestoft, L.: Metabolism of ethanol and fructose in the isolated perfused pig liver. Eur. J. Biochem. 33: 87–97 (1973).

Davenport, H.W.: Ethanol damage to canine oxyntic glandular mucosa. Proc. Soc. Exp. Biol. Med. 126: 657–662 (1967).

Davidson, M.B.; Bozarth, W.R.; Challoner, D.R. and Goodner, C.J.: Phenformin, hypoglycemia and lactic acidosis. New Eng. J. Med. 275: 886–888 (1966).

Davis, A.E. and Pirola, R.C.: The effects of ethyl alcohol on pancreatic exocrine function. Med. J. Aust. 2: 757–760 (1966).

Dayton, P.G. and Perel, S.M.: Physiological and physicochemical bases of drug interaction in man. Ann. N.Y. Acad. Sci. 179: 67–87 (1972).

De Carli, L.M. and Lieber, C.S.: Fatty liver in the rat after prolonged intake of ethanol with a nutritionally adequate new liquid diet. J. Nutr. 91: 331–336 (1967).

Deitrich, R.A.; Hellerman, L. and Wein, J.: Diphosphopyridine nucleotide-linked aldehyde dehydrogenase. I. Specificity and sigma-rho function. J. Biol. Chem. 237: 560–564 (1962).

De Marco, T.J. and Levine, R.R.: Role of the lymphatics in the intestinal absorption and distribution of drugs. J. Pharmacol. Exper. Therap. 169: 142–151 (1969).

Dinoso, V.P.; Chey, W.Y.; Braverman, S.; Rosen, A.P.; Ottenberg, D. and Lorber, S.H.: Gastric secretion and gastric mucosal morphology in chronic alcoholics. Arch. Int. Med. 130: 715–720 (1972).

Dobbins, W.O.; Rollins, E.L.; Brooks, S.G. and Fallon, H.J.: A quantitative morphological analysis of ethanol effect on rat liver. Gastroenterology 62: 1020–1033 (1972).

Douglas, J.F.; Ludwig, B.J. and Smith, N.: Studies on the metabolism of meprobamate. Proc. Soc. Exp. Biol. Med. 112: 436–438 (1963).

Dreisbach, R.H.: Handbook of poisoning, 4th ed. (Lange Medical Publications, Los Altos, California 1963).

Drum, D.P.; Harrison, J.H.; Li, T.-K.; Bethune, J.L. and Vallee, B.L.: Structural and functional zinc in horse liver alcohol dehydrogenase. Proc. Nat. Acad. Sci. U.S.A. 57: 1434–1440 (1967).

Edwards, J.A. and Evans, D.A.P.: Ethanol metabolism in subjects possessing typical and atypical liver alcohol dehydrogenase. Clin. Pharmacol. Therap. 8: 824–830 (1967).

Elmslie, R.G. and Harvey, N.: Alcohol absorption rate from different parts of the gut. Quart. J. Stud. Alc. 29: 308–312 (1967).

Elwin, C.E.: Stimulation of gastric acid secretion by irrigation of the antrum with some aliphatic alcohols. Acta Physiol. Scand. 75: 1–11 (1969a).

Elwin, C.E.: Some factors influencing the stimulatory effect of ethanol on gastric acid secretion during antrum application. Acta Physiol. Scand. 75: 12–27 (1969b).

Eriksson, K.: Behavioral and physiological differences among rat strains especially selected for their alcohol consumption. Ann. N.Y. Acad. Sci. 197: 32–41 (1972).

Ernster, L. and Lee, C.P.: Biological oxidoreductions. Ann. Rev. Biochem. 33: 729–788 (1964).

Evans, D.A.P.; Manley, K.A. and McKusick, V.C.: Genetic control of isoniazid metabolism in man. Brit. Med. J. 2: 485–491 (1960).

Feinman, L. and Lieber, C.S.: Hepatic collagen metabolism: effect of alcohol consumption in rats and baboons. Science 176: 795 (1972).

Feinman, L. and Lieber, C.S.: Liver disease in alcoholism; Ch. 9, in Kissin and Begleiter, The Biology of Alcoholism, vol. 3: Clinical Pathology (Plenum Press, New York and London 1974).

Fenna, D.; Mix, L.; Schaefer, O. and Gilbert, J.A.L.: Ethanol metabolism in various racial groups. Can. Med. Ass. 105: 472–475 (1971).

Ferguson, J.K.W.: A new drug for alcoholism treatment. Can. Med. Ass. J. 74: 793–795 (1956).

Ferguson, M.M.: Observations on the histochemical distribution of alcohol dehydrogenase. Quart. J. Micros. Sci. 106: 289–297 (1965).

Ferguson, M.M.; Baillie, A.M.; Calman, K.C. and McK. Hart, D.: Histochemical distribution of alcohol dehydrogenases in endocrine tissue. Nature 210: 1277–1279 (1966).

Figueroa, R.B. and Klotz, A.P.: Alterations of alcohol dehydrogenase and other hepatic enzymes following oral alcohol intoxication. Am. J. Clin. Nutr. 11: 235–239 (1962).

Fischer, H.D.: Der Einfluss von Barbituraten auf die Entgiftungsgeschwindigkeit des Äthanols. Biochem. Pharmacol. 11: 307–314 (1962).

Fisher, L.: Saregen wampforgiftning. Svensk Tandlakare – Tidskrift. 42: 2513–2515 (1945).

Fondal, E. and Kochakian, C.D.: In vitro effect of ethyl alcohol on respiration of rat liver and kidney slices. Proc. Soc. Exp. Biol. Med. 77: 823–824 (1951).

Formiller, M. and Cohon, M.S.: Coumarin and indanedione anticoagulants: potentiators and antagonists. Am. J. Hosp. Pharm. 26: 574–582 (1969).

Forney, R.B. and Harger, R.N.: Toxicology of ethanol. Ann. Rev. Pharmacol. 9: 379–392 (1969).

Forney, R.B. and Hughes, F.W.: Combined Effects of Alcohol and Other Drugs (C.C. Thomas, Springfield, Illinois 1968).

Forney, R.B. and Hughes, F.W.: Interaction between alcohol and psychopharmacologic drugs; in International Encyclopedia of Pharmacology and Therapy. Section 20, 'Alcohols and Derivatives', vol. II. pp.445–464 (Pergamon Press, Oxford and New York 1970).

Forsander, O.: Influence of the metabolism of ethanol on the lactate pyruvate ratio of rat liver slices. Biochem. J. 98: 244–247 (1966).

Forsander, O.A.: Influence of ethanol on the redox state of the liver. Quart. J. Stud. Alc. 31: 550–570 (1970).

Forsander, O. and Räihä, N.: Metabolites produced in the liver during alcohol oxidation. J. Biol. Chem. 235: 34–36 (1960).

Forsander, O.A.; Räihä, N. and Suomalainen, H.: Alkoholoxydation und Bildung von Acetoacetat in normaler und glycogenarmer intakter Rattenleber. Hoppe-Seyler's Ztschr. Physiol. Chem. 312: 243–248 (1958).

Forsander, O.; Räihä, N. and Suomalainen, H.: Oxydation des Äthylalkohols in isolierter Leber und isoliertem Hinterkörper der Ratte. Hoppe-Seyler's Ztschr. Physiol. Chem. 318: 1–5 (1960).

Forsander, O.A.; Räihä, N.; Salaspuro, M. and Maenpaa, P.: Influence of ethanol on the liver metabolism of fed and starved rats. Biochem. J. 94: 259–265 (1965).

Fouts, J.R. and Rogers, L.A.: Morphological changes in the liver accompanying stimulation of microsomal drug metabolising enzyme activity by phenobarbital chlordane, benzpyrene or methylcholanthrene in rats. J. Pharmacol. Exp. Therap. 147: 112–119 (1965).

French, S.W.: Acute and chronic toxicity of alcohol; Ch. 14 in Kissin and Begleiter, The Biology of Alcoholism, vol. 1: Biochemistry (Plenum Press, New York 1971).

Friedman, P.J. and Cooper, J.R.: The role of alcohol dehydrogenase in the metabolism of chloral hydrate. J. Pharmacol. Exper. Therap. 129: 373–376 (1960).

Fuge, C.A.: Treatment of poisoning by antidepressant drugs. Brit. Med. J. 2: 108 (1967).

Fuller, G.C.; Bousquet, W.F. and Miya, T.S.: Effect of cold exposure on drug action and hepatic drug metabolism in the rat. Toxicol. App. Pharmacol. 23: 10–19 (1972).

Fuhrman, G.J. and Fuhrman, F.A.: Effects of temperature on the action of drugs. Ann. Rev. Pharmacol. 1: 65–78 (1961).

Fujita, T. and Mannering, G.J.: Electron transport components of hepatic microsomes. J. Biol. Chem. 248: 8150–8156 (1973).

Furner, R.L. and Feller, D.D.: The influence of starvation upon hepatic drug metabolism in rats, mice and guinea pigs. Proc. Soc. Exp. Biol. Med. 137: 816–819 (1971).

Furner, R.L.; Gram, T.E. and Stitzel, R.E.: The influence of age, sex and drug treatment on microsomal drug metabolism in four rat strains. Biochem. Pharmacol. 18: 1635–1641 (1969).

Galambos, J.T. and Shapira, R.: Natural history of alcoholic hepatitis. IV. Glycosamino-glycuronans and collagen in the hepatic tissue. J. Clin. Invest. 52: 2952–2962 (1973).

Garner, R.C. and McLean, A.E.M.: Increased susceptibility to carbon tetrachloride poisoning in the rat after pretreatment with oral phenobarbitone. Biochem. Pharmacol. 18: 645–650 (1969).

Gessner, P.K. and Dien, L.H.: Kinetics of in vivo inhibition of ethanol by trichloroethanol and chloral hydrate (Abstract), in Proceedings Fourth International Congress of Pharmacology, p.372 (1969).

Gelboin, H.V.: Mechanisms of induction of drug metabolism enzymes; in La Du, Mandel and Way, Fundamentals of Drug Metabolism and Drug Disposition (Williams and Wilkins, Baltimore 1971).

Gielen, J.E. and Nebert, D.W.: Microsomal hydroxylase induction in liver cell culture by phenobarbital, polycyclic hydrocarbons, and p,p-DDT. Science 172: 167–169 (1971).

Gillette, J.R.: Metabolism of drugs and other foreign compounds by enzymatic mechanisms. Progress in Drug Research 6: 13–73 (1963).

Gillette, J.R.; Davis, D.C. and Sasame, H.A.; Cytochrome P-450 and its role in drug metabolism. Ann. Rev. Pharmacol. 12: 57–84 (1972).

Goldberg, L.: Effects of ethanol in the central nervous system; in Popham, Alcohol and Alcoholism (University of Toronto Press, 1970).

Goldberg, L. and Rydberg, U.: Inhibition of ethanol metabolism in vivo by administration of pyrazole. Biochem. Pharmacol. 18: 1749–1762 (1969).

Goldstein, D.B. and Nandita, P.: Alcohol dependence produced in mice by inhalation of ethanol: grading the withdrawal reaction. Science 172: 288–290 (1971).

Goodman, D.S. and Deykin, D.: Fatty acid ester formation during ethanol metabolism in vivo. Proc. Soc. Exp. Biol. Med. 113: 65–67 (1963).

Gordon, E.R.: The utilisation of ethanol by the isolated perfused liver. Can. J. Physiol. Pharmacol. 46: 609–616 (1968).

Gordon, E.R.: The effect of chronic consumption of ethanol on the redox state of the rat liver. Can. J. Biochem. 50: 949–957 (1972).

Gram, R.L.; Juchau, M.R. and Fouts, J.R.: Differences in hepatic drug metabolism in various rabbit strains before and after pretreatment with phenobarbital. Proc. Soc. Exp. Biol. Med. 118: 872–875 (1965).

Greenberg, L.A.: The appearance of some congeners of alcoholic beverages and their metabolites in the blood. Quart. J. Stud. Alc., Supp. 5: 20–25 (1970).

Greenberger, N.J.; Cohen, R.B. and Isselbacher, K.J.: The effect of chronic ethanol administration on liver alcohol dehydrogenase activity in the rat. Lab. Invest. 14: 264–271 (1965).

Greenblatt, D.J. and Greenblatt, M.: Which drug for alcohol withdrawal? J. Clin. Pharmacol. 12: 429–431 (1972).

Grell, E.H.; Jacobsen, K.B. and Murphy, J.B.: Alcohol dehydrogenase in Drosophila melanogaster: isoenzymes and genetic variants. Science 149: 80–82 (1965).

Griffaton, G. and Lowy, R.: Oxydation de l'éthanol in vitro par un homogénat de foie de rat. Comp. Rend. Soc. Biol. 158: 998–1003 (1964).

Grunnet, N.: Oxidation of acetaldehyde by rat-liver mitochondria in relation to ethanol oxidation and the transport of reducing equivalents across the mitochondrial membrane. Eur. J. Biochem. 35: 236–243 (1973).

Haag, H.B.; Finnegan, J.K.; Larson, P.S. and Smith, R.B.: Studies on the acute toxicity and irritating properties of the congeners in whisky. Toxicol. Appl. Pharmacol. 1: 618–627 (1959).

Haggard, H.W. and Greenberg, L.A.: Studies on the absorption, distribution and elimination of alcohol. V. The influence of glycocol upon the absorption of alcohol. J. Pharmacol. Exp. Therap. 68: 482–491 (1940).

Hald, J. and Jacobsen, E.: A drug sensitizing the organism to ethyl alcohol. Lancet 2: 1001 (1948a).

Hald, J. and Jacobsen, E.: The formation of acetaldehyde in the organism after ingestion of antabuse (tetraethylthiuram-disulfide) and alcohol. Acta Pharmacol. Toxicol. 4: 305–310 (1948b).

Hald, J.; Jacobsen, E. and Larsen, V.: The antabuse effect of some compounds related to antabuse and cyanamide. Acta Pharmacol. Toxicol. 8: 329–337 (1952).

Halstead, C.H.; Robles, E.A. and Mezey, E.: Decreased jejunal uptake of labeled folic acid (^{3}H-PGA) in alcoholic patients: roles of alcohol and nutrition. New Eng. J. Med. 285: 701–706 (1971).

Hanzlick, P.J. and Collins, R.J.: Quantitative studies on the gastrointestinal absorption of drugs. III. The absorption of alcohol. J. Pharmacol. Exp. Therap. 5: 185–191 (1913).

Harger, R.N. and Hulpieu, H.R.: The pharmacology of alcohol; Ch. 2, in Thompson, Alcoholism (C.C. Thomas, Springfield, Illinois 1956).

Harris, I.: Structure and catalytic activity of alcohol dehydrogenase. Nature 203: 30–34 (1964).

Harrop, G.A. and Benedict, E.M.: Acute methyl alcohol poisoning associated with acidosis. J. Am. Med. Ass. 74: 25 (1920).

Hart, L.G. and Fouts, J.R.: Studies on the possible mechanisms by which chlordane stimulates hepatic microsomal drug metabolism in the rat. Biochem. Pharmacol. 14: 263–272 (1965).

Hassinen, I.: Acetoin as a metabolite of ethanol. Acta Physiol. Scand. 57: 135–143 (1963).

Hassinen, I.: Hydrogen transfer into mitochondria in the metabolism of ethanol. I. Oxidation of the extramitochondrial reduced nicotinamide-adenine dinucleotide 45: 35–45 (1967).

Hassinen, I.E. and Ylikahri, R.H.: Mixed function oxidase and ethanol metabolism in perfused rat liver. Science 176: 1435–1437 (1972).

Hasumura, Y.; Teschke, R. and Lieber, C.S.: Increased carbon tetrachloride hepatotoxicity and its mechanism, after chronic ethanol consumption. Gastroenterology 66: 415–422 (1974).

Hatfield, G.K.; Miya, T.S. and Bousquet, W.F.: Ethanol tolerance and ethanol-drug interactions in the rat. Toxicol. Appl. Pharmacol. 23: 459–469 (1972).

Hawkins, R.D. and Kalant, H.: The metabolism of ethanol and its metabolic effects. Pharmacol. Rev. 24: 67–157 (1972).

Hawkins, R.D.; Kalant, H. and Khanna, J.M.: Effects of chronic intake of ethanol on rate of ethanol metabolism. Can. J. Physiol. Pharmacol. 44: 241–257 (1966).

Hayaishi, O.: Oxygenases; in Hayaishi, Enzyme Mechanisms (University Park Press, New York 1962).

Heim, F.; Ammon, H.P.T.; Estler, C.-J. and Mikschiczek, D.: Funktion und Stoffwechsel des Gehirns unter Einwirkung neidriger Alkoholkonzentrationen. Med. Pharmacol. Exp. 13: 361–370 (1965).

Hernandez, P.H.; Gillette, J.R. and Mazel, P.: Studies on the mechanism of action of mammalian hepatic azoreductase. I. Azoreductase activity of reduced nicotinamide adenine dinucleotide phosphate-cytochrome β reductase. Biochem. Pharmacol. 16: 1859–1875 (1967).

Hillbom, M.E.: Effect of ethanol on sorbitol metabolism in rats. Scand. J. Clin. Lab. Invest. 21, Suppl. 101: 18–19 (1968).

Hillbom, M.E. and Lindros, K.O.: Metabolic interaction of ethanol and sorbitol in relation to redox state of liver cytosol in hypo-, hyper-, and euthyroid rats. Metabolism 20: 843–849 (1971).

Hildebrandt, A. and Estabrook, R.W.: Evidence for the participation of cytochrome b_5 in hepatic microsomal mixed-function oxidation reactions. Arch. Biochem. Biophys. 143: 66–79 (1971).

Hine, C.H.; Burbridge, T.N.; Macklin, E.A.; Anderson, H.H. and Simon, A.: Some aspects of the human pharmacology of tetraethylthiuram disulphide (Antabuse) – alcohol reactions. J. Clin. Invest. 31: 317–325 (1952).

Hogben, C.A.M.; Schanker, L.S.; Tocco, D.J. and Brodie, B.B.: Absorption of drugs from the stomach. II. The human. J. Pharmacol. Exper. Therap. 120: 540–545 (1957).

Hollister, L.E.: Adverse reactions to drugs. Postgrad. Med. 37: 94–99 (1965).

Holtzman, J.L. and Gillette, J.R.: The effect of phenobarbital on the turnover of microsomal phospholipid in male and female rats. J. Biol. Chem. 243: 3020–3028 (1968).

Holzer, H. and Schneider, S.: Zum Mechanismus der Beeinflussung der Alkoholoxydation in der Leber durch Fructose. Klin. Wschr. 33: 1006–1009 (1955).

Horvath, S.M. and Willard, P.W.: Effect of ethyl alcohol upon splanchnic hemodynamics. Proc. Soc. Exp. Biol. Med. 111: 295–298 (1962).

Hrycay, E.G. and O'Brien, P.J.: Cytochrome P-450 as a microsomal peroxidase utilizing a lipid peroxide substrate. Arch. Biochem. Biophys. 147: 14–27 (1971).

Humphrey, T.J.: Methanol poisoning: management of acidosis with combined haemodialysis and peritoneal dialysis. Med. J. Aust. 1: 833–835 (1974).

Huttered, F. and Bacchin, P.: Mucopolysaccharides in normal and cirrhotic liver in man. Fed. Proc. 27: 412 (1968).

Huttered, F.; Denk, H. and Bacchin, P.G.: Mechanism of cholestasis. I. Effect of bile acids on microsomal cytochrome P-450 dependent biotransformation system in vitro. Life Sci. 9: 877–887 (1970).

Iber, F.L.: Alcohol and the gastrointestinal tract. Gastroenterology 61: 120–123 (1971).

Imai, Y. and Sato, R.: Evidence for two forms of P-450 hemoprotein in microsomal membranes. Biochem. Biophys. Res. Comm. 23: 5–11 (1966).

Isbell, H. and Chrúsciel, T.L.: Dependence Liability of Non-narcotic Drugs (World Health Organisation, Geneva 1970).

Iseri, O.A.; Gottlieb, L.S. and Lieber, C.S.: The ultrastructure of ethanol induced fatty liver. Fed. Proc. 23: 579 (1964).

Iseri, O.A,; Lieber, C.S. and Gottlieb, L.S.: The ultrastructure of fatty liver induced by prolonged ethanol ingestion. Am. J. Path. 48: 535–555 (1966).

Ishii, H.; Joly, J.-G. and Lieber, C.S.: Effect of ethanol on the amount of enzyme activities of hepatic rough and smooth microsomal membranes. Biochim. Biophys. Acta 291: 411–420 (1973).

Israel, Y.; Khanna, J.M. and Lin, R.: Effect of 2,4-dinitrophenol on the rate of ethanol elimination in the rat in vivo. Biochem. J. 120: 447–448 (1970).

Isselbacher, K.J. and Carter, E.A.: Ethanol oxidation by liver microsomes: evidence against a separate and distinct enzyme system. Biochem. Biophys. Res. Comm. 39: 530–537 (1970).

Isselbacher, K.J. and Krane, S.M.: Studies on the mechanism of the inhibition of galactose oxidation by ethanol. J. Biol. Chem. 236: 2394–2398 (1961).

Jacobsen, E.: The pharmacology of antabuse (tetraethylthiuram disulphide). Brit. J. Addiction 47: 26–40 (1950).

Jacobsen, E.: The metabolism of ethyl alcohol. Pharmacol. Rev. 4: 107–135 (1952).

Jacobson, M.; Lu, A.Y.H.; Sernatinger, E.; West, S. and Kuntzman, R.: The effect of altering liver microsomal CO-binding hemoprotein composition on pentobarbital-induced anesthesia. Chemico-Biological Interactions 5: 183–189 (1972).

Jaffe, J.H.: Drug addiction and abuse; Ch. 16, in Goodman and Gilman, The Pharmacological Basis of Therapeutics, 4th ed. (The Macmillan Co., London 1970).

James, T.N. and Bear, E.S.: Effects of ethanol and acetaldehyde on the heart. Am. Heart J. 74: 242–255 (1967).

James, T.N. and Bear, E.S.: Cardiac effects of simple aliphatic aldehydes. J. Pharmacol. Exper. Therap. 163: 300–308 (1968).

Janz, D. and Schmidt, D.: Anti-epileptic drugs and failure of oral contraceptives. Lancet 1: 1113 (1974).

Jarvik, M.E.: Drugs used in the treatment of psychiatric disorders; Ch. 12, in Goodman and Gilman, The Pharmacological Basis of Therapeutics (The Macmillan Co., London and Toronto 1970).

Jaulmes, C.; Delga, J. and Gary Bobo, C.: Métabolisme de l'alcool chez les aminaux soumis à l'hibernation artificielle. Comp. Rend. Soc. Biol. 150: 1094–1101 (1956).

Jeejeebhoy, K.N.; Phillips, M.J.; Bruce-Robertson, A.; Ho, J. and Sodtke, U.: The acute effect of ethanol on albumin, fibrinogen and transferrin synthesis in the rat. Biochem. J. 126: 1111–1126 (1972).

Jefcoate, C.R.E.; Gaylor, J.L. and Calabrese, R.L.: Ligand interactions with cytochrome P-450. I. Binding of primary amines. Biochemistry 8: 3455–3463 (1969).

Jeliffe, R.W. and Blankenhorn, D.H.: Effect of phenobarbital on digitoxin metabolism. Clin. Res. 14: 160 (1961).

Jick, H.: Drugs — Remarkably Non Toxic. N. Engl. J. Med. 291: 824–828 (1974).

Joly, J.-G.; Ishii, H.; Teschke, R.; Hasumura, Y. and Lieber, C.S.: Effect of chronic ethanol feeding on the activities and submicrosomal distribution of reduced nicotinamide adenine dinucleotide phosphate (NADPH)–cytochrome P-450 reductase and the demethylases for aminopyrine and ethylmorphine. Biochem. Pharmacol. 22: 1532–1535 (1973).

Joly, J.-G.; Ishii, H. and Lieber, C.S.: Microsomal cyanide-binding cytochrome: Its role in hepatic etharol oxidation. Gastroenterology 62: 174 (1972).

Jörnvall, H.: Differences in E and S chains from iso-enzymes of horse liver alcohol dehydrogenase. Nature 225: 113–1134 (1970).

Jörnvall, H. and Harris, J.I.: Horse liver alcohol dehydrogenase: On the primary structure of the ethanol active isoenzyme. Eur. J. Biochem. 13: 565–576 (1970).

Kahonen, M.T.; Ylikahri, R.H. and Hassinen, I.: Ethanol metabolism in rats treated with ethyl-α-p-chlorophenoxyisobutyrate (Clofibrate). Life Sci. 10: 661–670 (1971).

Kalant, H.: Absorption, diffusion, distribution and elimination of ethanol: effects of biological membranes; Ch. 1, in Kissin and Begleiter, The Biology of Alcoholism, vol. 1 (Plenum Press, New York 1971).

Kalant, H.; Hawkins, R.D. and Watkin, G.S.: The effect of ethanol on the metabolic rate of rats. Can. J. Biochem. Physiol. 41: 2197–2203 (1963).

Kalant, H.; Khanna, J.M. and Loth, J.: Effect of chronic intake of ethanol on pyridine nucleotide levels in rat liver and kidney. Can. J. Physiol. Pharmacol. 48: 542–549 (1970).

Kalant, H.; Khanna, J.M. and Marshman, J.: Effect of chronic intake of ethanol on pentobarbital metabolism. J. Pharmacol. Exp. Therap. 175: 318–324 (1970).

Kaplan, N.O.; Ciotti, M.M. and Stolzenbach, F.E.: Reaction of pyridine nucleotide analogues with dehydrogenase. J. Biol. Chem. 221: 833–844 (1956).

Kaplan, H.L.; Forney, R.B.; Hughes, F.W. and Jain, N.C.: Chloral hydrate and alcohol metabolism in human subjects. J. For. Sci. 12: 295–304 (1967a).

Kaplan, H.L.; Forney, R.B.; Hughes, F.W.; Richards, A.B. and Jain, N.C.: Ethanol effects on chloral hydrate metabolism in mice. Toxicol. Appl. Pharmacol. 10: 387–394 (1967b).

Karasek, M.A. and Greenberg, D.M.: Studies on the properties of threonine aldolases J. Biol. Chem. 227: 191–205 (1957).

Kater, R.M.H.; Carulli, N. and Iber, F.L.: Differences in the rate of ethanol metabolism in recently drinking alcoholic and non-alcoholic subjects. Am. J. Clin. Nutr. 22: 1608–1617 (1969a).

Kater, R.M.H.; Roggin, G.; Tobon, F.; Zieve, P. and Iber, F.L.: Increased rate of clearance of drugs from the circulation of alcoholics. Am. J. Med. Sci. 258: 35–39 (1969b).

Kater, R.M.H.; Tobon, F. and Iber, F.L.: Increased rate of tolbutamide metabolism in alcoholic patients. J. Am. Med. Ass. 207: 363–365 (1969c)

Kater, R.M.H.; Zieve, P.; Tobon, F.; Roggin, C. and Iber, F.L.: Accelerated metabolism of drugs in alcoholics. Gastroenterology 56: 412 (1969).

Kato, R.: Sex difference in the activities of microsomal drug-metabolizing enzyme systems in relation to dietary protein. Japan. J. Pharmacol. 16: 221–223 (1966).

Kato, R.: Effect of administration of 3-aminotriazole on the activity of microsomal drug metabolising enzyme systems of rat liver. Japan. J. Pharmacol. 17: 56–63 (1967).

Kato, R. and Gillette, J.R.: Effect of starvation on NADPH-dependent enzymes in liver microsomes of male and female rats. J. Pharmacol. Exp. Therap. 150: 279–284 (1965).

Kato, R. and Takanaka, A.: Metabolism of drugs in old rats. II. Metabolism in vivo and effect of drugs in old rats. Japan. J. Pharmacol. 18: 389–396 (1968).

Keilin, D. and Hartree, E.F.: Properties of catalase. Catalysis of coupled oxidation of alcohols. Biochem. J. 39: 293–301 (1945).

Kelley, W.N.; Green, M.L.; Rosenbloom, F.M.; Henderson, J.F. and Seegmiller, J.E.: Hypoxanthine-guanine phosphoribosyltransferase deficiency in gout. Ann. Int. Med. 70: 155–206 (1969).

Khanna, J.M. and Kalant, H.: Metabolic interactions of ethanol and drugs. Proceedings of the Symposium on Biological Aspects of Alcohol (University of Texas Press, 1970).

Khanna, J.M.; Kalant, H. and Lin, G.: Metabolism of ethanol by rat liver microsomal enzymes. Biochem. Pharmacol. 19: 2493–2499 (1970).

Khanna, J.M.; Kalant, H. and Lin, G.: Effect of carbon tetrachloride treatment on ethanol metabolism. Biochem. Pharmacol. 20: 3269–3279 (1971).

Khanna, J.M.; Kalant, H. and Lin, G.: Significance in vivo of the increase in microsomal ethanol-oxidizing system after chronic administration of ethanol, phenobarbital and chlorcyclizine. Biochem. Pharmacol. 21: 2215–2226 (1972).

Khouw, L.B.; Burbridge, T.N. and Sutherland, V.C.: The inhibition of alcohol dehydrogenase. I. Kinetic studies. Biochim. Biophys. Acta 73: 173–185 (1963).

Kiessling, K.-H. and Pilstrom, L.: Effect of ethanol on rat liver. Enzymatic and histological studies of liver mitochondria. Quart. J. Stud. Alc. 27: 189–200 (1966).

Kinard, F.W.; Hay, M.G. and Nelson, G.H.: Effect of starvation on alcohol metabolism and hepatic enzyme activities in dogs. Quart. J. Stud. Alc. 21: 203–207 (1960).

Kissin, B.: The pharmacodynamics and natural history of alcoholism; Ch. 1, in Kissin and Begleiter, The Biology of Alcoholism, vol 3: Clinical Pathology (Plenum Press, New York 1974a).

Kissin, B.: Interactions of ethyl alcohol and other drugs; Ch. 4, in Kissin and Begleiter, The Biology of Alcoholism, vol. 3: Clinical Pathology (Plenum Press, New York 1974b).

Kissin, B. and Begleiter, H.: The Biology of Alcoholism, vol. 1: Biochemistry (Plenum Press, New York and London 1971).

Kissin, B. and Begleiter, H.: The Biology of Alcoholism, vol. 3: Clinical Pathology (Plenum Press, New York and London 1974).

Kissin, B.; Gross, M.M. and Schutz, I.: Correlation of urinary biogenic amines with sleep stages in chronic alcoholization and withdrawal; in Gross, Experimental Studies of Alcohol Intoxication and Withdrawal (Plenum Press, New York 1973).

Klassen, C.D.: Ethanol metabolism in rats after microsomal metabolizing enzyme induction. Proc. Soc. Exp. Biol. Med. 132: 1099–1102 (1969).

Klatskin, G.: The effect of ethyl alcohol on nitrogen excretion in the rat. Yale J. Biol. Med. 24: 124–143 (1961).

Klatskin, G.: Toxic and drug induced hepatitis; Ch. 14, in Schiff, Diseases of the Liver, 3rd ed. (J.B. Lippincott Co., Philadelphia 1969).

Klipstein, F.A.; Holdeman, L.V.; Corcino, J.J. and Moore, W.E.C.: Enteropathogenic intestinal bacteria in tropical sprue. Gastroenterology 64: 754 (1973).

Knapp, S. and Mandel, A.J.: Serotonin-biosynthesis systems of the brain. Science 177: 1209–1211 (1972).

Koen, A.L. and Shaw, C.R.: Retinol and alcohol dehydrogenases in retina and liver. Biochim. Biophys. Acta 128: 48–54 (1966).

Koivusalo, M. and Tarkkanen, A.: Alcohol dehydrogenase activities of retina and brain. Federation of the European Biochemical Societies, 6th Meeting, Madrid, Abstract of communications, p.75 (1969).

Kolmodin, B.; Azarnoff, D.L. and Sjöqvist, F.: Effect of environmental factors on drug metabolism: Decreased plasma half life of antipyrine in workers exposed to chlorinated insecticides. J. Clin. Pharmacol. Therap. 10: 638–642 (1969).

Kraemer, R.J. and Deitrich, R.A.: Isolation and characterization of human liver aldehyde dehydrogenase. J. Biol. Chem. 243: 6402–6408 (1968).

Krebs, H.A.: The cause of the specific dynamic action of foodstuffs. Arzneimittel-Forschung. 10: 369–373 (1960).

Krebs, H.A.: Role of the redox state of nicotinamide adenine dinucleotides in the regulation of metabolic processes. Nat. Cancer Inst. Monographs 27: 331–343 (1967).

Krebs, H.A. and Perkins, J.R.: The physiological role of liver alcohol dehydrogenase. Biochem. J. 118: 635–644 (1970).

Kreisberg, R.A.; Owen, W.C. and Siegal, A.M.: Hyperlactacidemia in man: ethanol-phenformin synergism. J. Clin. Endocr. 34: 29–35 (1972).

Kuntzman, R.; Jacobson, M. and Conney, A.H.: Effect of phenylbutazone on cortisol metabolism in man. Pharmacology 8: 195 (1966).

Kuriyama, Y.; Omura, T.; Siekevitz, P. and Palade, G.E.: Effect of phenobarbital on the synthesis and degradation of the components of rat liver microsomal membranes. J. Biol. Chem. 244: 2017–2026 (1969).

Kuriyama, K.; Rauscher, G.E. and Sze, P.Y.: Effect of acute and chronic administration of ethanol on 5-hydroxytryptamine turnover and tryptophan hydroxylase activity of the mouse brain. Brain Res. 26: 450–454 (1971).

La Du, B.N.: Pharmacogenetics. Med. Clin. N. Amer. 53: 839–855 (1969).

Lal, S.: Metronidazole in the treatment of alcoholism. Quart J. Stud. Alc. 30: 140–151 (1969).

Landauer, A.A.; Milner, G. and Patman, J.: Alcohol and amitriptyline effects on skills related to driving behaviour. Science 163: 1467–1468 (1969).

Landauer, A.A. and Milner, G.: Desipramine and imipramine, alone and together with alcohol in relation to driving safety. Pharmakopsych. Neuro-psychopharmakol. 4: 265–275 (1971).

Lane, B.P. and Lieber, C.S.: Effects of butylated hydroxytoluene (BHT) on the ultra-structure of rat hepatocytes. Lab. Invest. 16: 342–348 (1967).

Larsen, J.A.: Extrahepatic metabolism of ethanol in man. Nature 184: 1236 (1959).

Lasagna, L.: The diseases drugs cause. Perspectives in Biology and Medicine 7: 457–470 (1964).

Latham, A.N.; Millbank, L.; Richens, A. and Rowe, D.J.F.: Liver enzyme induction by anticonvulsant drugs, and its relationship to disturbed calcium and folic acid metabolism. J. Clin. Pharmacol. 13: 337–342 (1973).

Läuppi, E.: Antabusähnliche Wirkung von Irgapyrin. Schweiz. Med. Wschr. 84: 1281–1287 (1954).

Leake, C.D. and Silverman, M.: Alcoholic Beverages in Clinical Medicine (Year Book Medical Publishers, Chicago 1966).

Leake, C.D. and Silverman, M.: The chemistry of alcoholic beverages; Ch. 17, in Kissin and Begleiter, The Biology of Alcoholism, vol. 1: Biochemistry (Plenum Press, Oxford and New York 1971).

Learoyd, B.M.: The effect of sedatives on metabolic rate during alcohol withdrawal. Quart. J. Stud. Alc. 33: 22–32 (1972).

Le Breton, E.: Signification physiologique de l'oxydation de l'alcool dans l'organisme. Ann. Physiol. Physicochim. Biol. 12: 369–457 (1936).

Lefevre, A.F.; De Carli, L.M. and Lieber, C.S.: Effect of ethanol on cholesterol and bile acid metabolism. J. Lipid Res. 13: 48–55 (1972).

Leloir, L.F. and Munoz, J.M.: Ethyl alcohol metabolism in animal tissues. Biochem. J. 32: 299–307 (1938).

Levin, W. and Kuntzman, R.: Biphasic decrease in radioactive hemoprotein from rat liver CO-binding particles: Effect of 3-methylcholanthrene. J. Biol. Chem. 244: 3671–3676 (1969).

Levi, A.J.; Sherlock, S. and Walker, D.: Phenylbutazone and isoniazid metabolism in patients with liver disease in relation to previous drug therapy. Lancet 1: 1275–1279 (1968).

Levy, G.: Drug biotransformation interactions in man: non-narcotic analgesics. Ann. N.Y. Acad. Sci. 179: 32–42 (1971).

Lieber, C.S.: New pathway of ethanol metabolism in the liver. Gastroenterology 59: 930–937 (1970).

Lieber, C.S.: Metabolism of ethanol and alcoholism: Racial and acquired factors. Ann. Int. Med. 76: 326–327 (1972a).

Lieber, C.S.: Ethanol metabolism and biochemical aspects of alcohol tolerance and dependence; in Mule and Brill, Chemical and Biological Aspects of Drug Dependence (Chemical Rubber Company Press, Cleveland, Ohio 1972b).

Lieber, C.S.: Progress in hepatology. Hepatic and metabolic effects of alcohol (1966 to 1973). Gastroenterology 65: 821–846 (1973a).

Lieber, C.S.: Liver adaptation and injury in alcoholism. New Eng. J. Med. 288: 356–362 (1973b).

Lieber, C.S.: Effects of ethanol upon lipid metabolism. Lipids 9: 103–116 (1974).

Lieber, C.S. and Davidson, C.S.: Some metabolic effects of ethyl alcohol. Am. J. Med. 33: 319–327 (1962).

Lieber, C.S. and De Carli, L.M.: Ethanol oxidation by hepatic microsomes: Adaptive increase after ethanol feeding. Science 162: 917–918 (1968).

Lieber, C.S. and De Carli, L.M.: Hepatic microsomal ethanol-oxidizing system: in vitro characteristics and adaptive properties in vivo. J. Biol. Chem. 245: 2505–2512 (1970a).

Lieber, C.S. and De Carli, L.M.: Reduced nicotinamide-adenine dinucleotide phosphate oxidase: activity enhanced by ethanol consumption. Science 170: 78–80 (1970b).

Lieber, C.S. and De Carli, L.M.: Effect of drug administration on the activity of the hepatic microsomal ethanol oxidizing system. Life Sci. 9 (Part II): 267–276 (1970c).

Lieber, C.S. and De Carli, L.M.: Quantitative relationship between amount of dietary fat and severity of alcoholic fatty liver. Am. J. Clin. Nutr. 23: 474–478 (1970d).

Lieber, C.S. and De Carli, L.M.: The role of the hepatic microsomal ethanol oxidizing system (MEOS) for ethanol metabolism in vivo. J. Pharmacol. Exp. Therap. 181: 279–287 (1972).

Lieber, C.S. and De Carli, L.M.: The significance and characterization of hepatic microsomal ethanol oxidation in the liver. Drug. Metab. Disp. 1: 428–440 (1973a).

Lieber, C.S. and De Carli, L.M.: Ethanol dependence and tolerance: a nutritionally controlled experimental model in the rat. Res. Comm. Chem. Path. Pharmacol. 6: 983–991 (1973b).

Lieber, C.S. and De Carli, L.M.: An experimental model of alcohol feeding and liver injury in the baboon. J. Med. Prim. 3: 153–163 (1974).

Lieber, C.S. and Rubin, E.: Alcoholic fatty liver in man on a high protein and low fat diet. Am. J. Med. 44: 200–207 (1968).

Lieber, C.S.; De Carli, L.M. and Gang, H.: Hepatic effects of longterm ethanol consumption in primates; in Goldsmith and Moor-Jankowski, Proceedings of the Third Conference on Experimental Medicine and Surgery in Primates, vol. 3 (S. Karger, Basel 1973).

Lieber, C.S.; Jones, D.P.; Losowsky, M.S. and Davidson, C.S.: Interrelation of uric acid and ethanol metabolism in man. J. Clin. Invest. 41: 1863–1870 (1962).

Lieber, C.S.; Rubin, E. and De Carli, L.M.: Hepatic microsomal ethanol oxidizing system (MEOS); differentiation from alcohol dehydrogenase and NADPH oxidase. Biochem. Biophys. Res. Comm. 40: 858–865 (1970).

Lieber, C.S.; Rubin, E.; De Carli, L.M.; Misra, P. and Gang, H.: Effects of pyrazole on hepatic function and structure. Lab. Invest. 22: 615–621 (1970).

Lieber, C.S.; Rubin, E. and De Carli, L.M.: Effects of ethanol on lipid, uric acid, intermediary, and drug metabolism, including the pathogenesis of the alcoholic fatty liver; Ch. 8, in Kissin and Begleiter, The Biology of Alcoholism, vol. 1: Biochemistry (Plenum Press, New York 1971).

Lieber, C.S.; Spritz, N. and De Carli, L.M.: Accumulation of triglycerides in heart and kidney after ethanol ingestion. J. Clin. Invest. 45: 1041 (1966).

Lin, G.; Kalant, H. and Khanna, J.M.: Catalase involvement in microsomal ethanol-oxidizing system. Biochem. Pharmacol. 21: 3305–3308 (1972).

Lockett, M.F. and Milner, G.: Combining the antidepressant drugs. Brit. Med. J. 1: 921–926 (1965).

Loewy, A.G. and Siekevitz, P.: Cell Structure and Function, 2nd ed. (Holt, Rinehart and Winston, Inc., New York 1969).

Lolli, G. and Greenberg, L.A.: The effect of insulin on the rate of disappearance of alcohol from the stomach. Quart. J. Stud. Alc. 3: 92–101 (1942).

Loomis, T.H.: Study of the rate of metabolism of ethyl alcohol with special reference to certain factors reported as influencing this rate. Quart. J. Stud. Alc. 11: 527–537 (1950).

Lowe, C.U. and Mosowich, L.: The paradoxical effect of alcohol on carbohydrate metabolism in four patients with liver glycogen disease. Pediatrics 35: 1005–1008 (1965).

Lu, A.Y.H. and Coon, M.J.: Role of hemoprotein P-450 in fatty acid ω-hydroxylation in a soluble enzyme system from liver microsomes. J. Biol. Chem. 243: 1331–1332 (1968).

Lu, A.Y.H.; Kuntzman, R.; West, S.; Jacobson, M. and Conney, A.H.: Reconstituted liver microsomal enzyme system that hydroxylates drugs, other foreign compounds, and endogenous substrates. II. Role of the cytochrome P-450 and P-448 fractions in drug and steroid hydroxylations. J. Biol. Chem. 247: 1727–1734 (1972).

Lüders, D.: Einfluss von Phenobarbital auf die Schilddrüsenfunktion bei Wistar- und Gunnratten. Z. Kinderheilkunde 113: 129–144 (1972).

Lundquist, F.: Enzymatic pathways of ethanol metabolism; in Trémolières, Encyclopedia of Alcohol and Alcoholism, vol. 1 (Pergamon Press, Oxford 1970).

Lundquist, F.; Fugman, U.; Rasmussen, H. and Svendsen, I.: The metabolism of acetaldehyde in mammalian tissues. Reactions in rat liver suspensions under aerobic conditions. Biochem. J. 84: 281–286 (1962a).

Lundquist, F.; Tygstrup, N.; Winkler, K.; Mellemgaard, K. and Munck-Petersen, S.: Ethanol metabolism and production of free acetate in the human liver. J. Clin. Invest. 41: 955–961 (1962b).

Lundquist, F.; Svendsen, I. and Petersen, P.H.: Metabolism of ethanol in rat liver suspensions. Biochem. J. 86: 119–124 (1963).

Lundsgaard, E.: Alcohol oxidation in the liver. Comp. Rend. Lab. Carlsberg Serie Chim. Clin. 22: 333–337 (1938).

Lutstorf, U.M. and Megnet, R.: Multiple forms of alcohol dehydrogenase in saccharomyces cerevisiae. Arch. Biochem. Biophys. 126: 933–944 (1968).

Lutstorf, U.M. and Von Wartburg, J.-P.: Hybridization of horse liver alcohol dehydrogenase isoenzymes. Federation of European Biochemical Societies. Sixth meeting, Abstracts of communications, Madrid (1969).

MacDonald, M.G.; Robinson, D.S.; Sylwester, D. and Jaffe, J.J.: The effects of phenobarbital, chloral betaine and glutethimide administration on warfarin plasma levels and hypoprothrombinaemic responses in man. Clin. Pharmacol. Therap. 10: 80–84 (1969).

Maddrey, W.C. and Boyer, J.L.: The acute and chronic effects of ethanol administration on bile secretion in the rat. Journal of Laboratory and Clinical Medicine 82: 215–225 (1973).

Makar, A.B.; Tephly, T.R. and Mannering, G.J.: Methanol metabolism in the monkey. Mol. Pharmacol. 4: 471–483 (1968).

Mallov, S. and Baesl, T.J.: Effect of ethanol on rates of elimination and metabolism of zoxazolamine, hexobarbital and warfarin sodium in the rat. Biochemical Pharmacology 21: 1667–1678 (1972).

Mannering, G.J.: Significance of stimulation and inhibition of drug metabolism; in Burger, Selected Pharmacological Testing Methods (Marcel Dekker, New York 1968).

Mannering, G.J.: Microsomal enzyme systems which catalyze drug metabolism; Ch. 12, in La Du, Mandel and Way, Fundamentals of Drug Metabolism and Drug Disposition (Williams and Wilkins, Baltimore 1971).

Marconi, J.; Solari, G. and Gaete, S.: Comparative clinical study of the effects of disulfiram and calcium carbimide. Quart. J. Stud. Alc. 22: 46–51 (1961).

Mardones, J.: The alcohols; in Root and Hofmann, Physiological Pharmacology, vol. 1 (Academic Press, New York 1963).

Marshall, E.K. and Owens, A.H.: Absorption, excretion and metabolic fate of chloral hydrate and trichloroethanol. Bull. Johns Hopkins Hosp. 95: 1–18 (1954).

Mason, H.S.: Oxidases. Annual Review of Biochemistry 34: 595–634 (1965).

Masters, A.B.: Delayed death in imipramine poisoning. British Medical Bulletin 2: 866–867 (1967).

Maxwell, J.D.; Hunter, J.; Stewart, D.A.; Ardeman, S. and Williams, R.: Folate deficiency after anticonvulsant drugs: An effect of hepatic enzyme induction? Br. Med. J. 1: 297–299 (1972).

McKenzie, J.C.: Social implications of alcohol consumption. Proc. Nutr. Soc. 31: 99–106 (1972).

McManus, I.R.; Contag, A.O. and Olson, R.E.: Studies on the identification and origin of ethanol on mammalian tissues. J. Biol. Chem. 241: 349–356 (1966).

Meldolesi, J.: On the significance of the hypertrophy of the smooth endoplasmic reticulum in liver cells after administration of drugs. Biochem. Pharmacol. 16: 125–131 (1967).

Mellanby, E.: Alcohol: Its Absorption into and Disappearance from the Blood under Different Conditions. Medical Research Committee Special Report Series No. 31, London, His Majesty's Stationery Office (1919).

Melmon, K.L.: Preventable drug reactions – causes and cures. New Eng. J. Med. 284: 1361–1368 (1971).

Mezey, E. and Robles, E.A.: Effects of phenobarbital administration on rates of ethanol clearance and on ethanol-oxidizing enzymes in man. Gastroenterology 66: 248–253 (1974).

Mezey, E. and Tobon, F.: Rates of ethanol clearance and activities of the ethanol-oxidizing enzymes in chronic alcoholic patients. Gastroenterology 61: 707–715 (1971).

Mezey, E.; Jow, E.; Slavin, R.E. and Tobon, F.: Pancreatic function and intestinal absorption in chronic alcoholism. Gastroenterology 59: 657–664 (1970).

Mezey, E.; Potter, J. and Reed, W.D.: Ethanol oxidation by a component of liver microsomes rich in cytochrome P-450. J. Biol. Chem. 248: 1183–1187 (1973).

Milner, G.: Amitriptyline – potentiation of alcohol. Lancet 1: 222–223 (1967).

Milner, G.: Drugs and Driving; In Avery, Monographs on Drugs, vol. 1 (ADIS Press, Sydney 1972).

Misra, P.S.; Lefevre, A.; Ishii, H.; Rubin, E. and Lieber, C.S.: Increase of ethanol, meprobamate and pentobarbital metabolism after chronic ethanol administration in man and in rats. Am. J. Med. 51: 346–351 (1971).

Mistilis, S.P. and Garske, A.: Induction of alcohol dehydrogenase in liver and gastrointestinal tract. Aust. Ann. Med. 18: 227–231 (1969).

Mitchell, E.H.: Use of citrated calcium carbimide in alcoholism. J. Am. Med. Ass. 168: 2008–2009 (1958).

Mitchell, H.H.: The food value of ethyl alcohol. J. Nutr. 10: 311–335 (1935).

Mitchell, H. and Curzon, E.G.: The food value of ethyl alcohol. Quart. J. Stud. Alc. 1: 227–245 (1940).

Morin, Y. and Daniel, P.: Quebec beer-drinkers' cardiomyopathy: etiological considerations. Canad. Med. Ass. J. 97: 926–928 (1967).

Morini, I.: Su alcuni casi di avvelenamento da glicol etilenico commerciale. Minerva Medica 1: 72–77 (1954).

Morrison, G.R. and Brock, F.E.: Quantitative measurement of alcohol dehydrogenase activity within the liver lobule of rats after prolonged ethanol ingestion. J. Nutr. 92: 286–292 (1967).

Moser, R.H.: Iatrogenic disorders. Milit. Med. 135: 619–630 (1970).

Moser, K.; Papenberg, J. and Von Wartburg, J.-P.: Heterogänitet und Organverteilung der Alkoholdehydrogenase bei verschiedenen Spezies. Enzymol. Biol. Clin. 9: 447–458 (1969).

Moses, S.W.; Levin, S.; Chayoth, R. and Steinitz, K.: Enzyme induction in a case of glycogen storage disease. Pediatrics 28: 111–121 (1966).

Mould, G.P.; Curry, S.H. and Binns, T.B.: Interaction of glutethimide and phenobarbitone with ethanol in man. J. Pharm. Pharmacol. 24: 894–899 (1972).

Mourad, N. and Woronick, C.L.: Crystallization of human liver alcohol dehydrogenase. Arch. Biochem. Biophys. 121: 431–439 (1967).

Mueller, G.C. and Miller, J.A.: The reductive cleavage of 4-demethylamino-azobenzene by fat liver: the intracellular distribution of the enzyme system and its requirement for triphosphopyridine nucleotide. J. Biol. Chem. 180: 1125–1136 (1949).

Mumford, J.P.: Drugs affecting oral contraceptives. Lancet 1: 333–334 (1974).

Murphree, H.B.: The importance of congeners in the effects of alcoholic beverages; in Israel and Mardones, Biological Basis of Alcoholism (John Wiley and Sons, New York 1971).

Murphree, H.B.; Greenberg, L.A. and Carroll, R.B.: Neuropharmacological effects of substances other than ethanol in alcoholic beverages. Fed. Proc. 26: 1468–1473 (1967).

Musacchio, J.M.; Bhagat, B.; Jackson, C.J. and Kopin, I.J.: The effect of disulfiram on the restoration of the response to tyramine by dopamine and methyldopa in the reserpine-treated cat. J. Pharmacol. Exp. Therap. 152: 293–297 (1966).

Nair, V.; Brown, T.; Bau, D. and Siegel, S.: Hypothalamic regulation of hepatic hexobarbital metabolizing enzyme system. Eur. J. Pharmacol. 9: 31–40 (1970).

Negelein, E. and Wulff, H.J.: Diphosphopyridinproteid, Alcohol, Acetaldehyd. Biochem. Z. 293: 351–389 (1937).

Newman, H.W. and Mehrtens, W.G.: Effect of intravenous injection of ethyl alcohol on gastric secretion in man. Proc. Soc. Exp. Biol. Med. 30: 145–148 (1932).

Newsome, W.H. and Rattray, J.B.M.: The enzymatic esterification of ethanol with fatty acids. Can. J. Biochem. 43: 1223–1235 (1965).

Nikkilä, E.A. and Ojala, L.: Role of L-alpha-glycerophosphate and triglyceride synthesis in production of fatty liver by ethanol. Proc. Exp. Biol. Med. 113: 814–817 (1963).

Nyberg, A.; Schuberth, J. and Anggard, L.: On the intracellular distribution of catalase and alcohol dehydrogenase. Acta Chemica Scand. 7: 1170–1172 (1953).

Ohnhaus, E.E.; Thorgeirsson, S.S.; Davies, D.S. and Breckenridge, A.: Changes in liver blood flow during enzyme induction. Biochem. Pharmacol. 20: 2561–2570 (1971).

Oppenheimer, J.H.; Bernstein, G. and Surks, M.I.: Increased thyroxine turnover and thyroidal function after stimulation of hepatocellular binding of thyroxine by phenobarbital. J. Clin. Invest. 47: 1399–1406 (1968).

O'Reilly, R.A.: The second reported kindred with inherited resistance to oral anticoagulant drugs. New Eng. J. Med. 282: 1448–1451 (1970).

Orme-Johnson, W.H. and Ziegler, D.M.: Alcohol mixed function oxidase activity of mammalian liver microsomes. Biochem. Biophys. Res. Comm. 21: 78–82 (1965).

Orrhenius, S. and Ernster, L.: Phenobarbital-induced synthesis of the oxidative demethylating enzymes of rat liver microsomes. Biochem. Biophys. Res. Comm. 16: 60–65 (1964).

Orrhenius, S. and Ericsson, J.L.E.: Enzyme-membrane relationship in phenobarbital induction of synthesis of drug metabolizing enzyme system and proliferation of endoplasmic membranes. J. Cell Biol. 28: 181–198 (1966).

Orrhenius, S.; Ericsson, J. and Ernster, L.: Phenobarbital-induced synthesis of the microsomal drug-metabolizing enzyme system and its relationship to the proliferation of endoplasmic membranes. J. Cell Biol. 25: 627–640 (1965).

Oshino, N.; Imai, Y. and Sato, R.: A function of cytochrome b_5 in fatty acid desaturation by rat liver microsomes. J. Biochem. 69: 155–167 (1971).

Oshino, N.; Oshino, R. and Chance, B.: The characteristics of the 'peroxidative' reaction of catalase in ethanol oxidation. Biochem. J. 131: 555–563 (1973).

Owen, N.V.; Griffing, W.J.; Hoffman, D.G.; Gibson, W.R. and Anderson, R.C.: Effects of dietary administration of 5-(3,4-dichlorophenyl)-5-ethylbarbituric acid (dichlorophenobarbital) to rats: emphasis on hepatic drug-metabolizing enzymes and morphology. Toxicol. App. Pharmacol. 18: 720–733 (1971).

Owens, A.H. and Marshall, E.K.: Further studies on the metabolic fate of chloral hydrate and trichloroethanol. Bulletin of the Johns Hopkins Hospital 97: 320–326 (1955).

Owens, A.H.; Marshall, E.K.; Broun, G.O.; Zubrod, K. and Lasagna, L.: A comparative evaluation of the hypnotic potency of chloral hydrate and trichloroethanol. Bulletin of the Johns Hopkins Hospital 96: 71–83 (1955).

Papenberg, J.; Von Wartburg, J.-P. and Aebi, H.: Metabolism of ethanol and fructose in the perfused rat liver. Enzym. Biol. Clin. 11: 237–250 (1970).

Park, S.K. and Brody, J.I.: Suppression of immunity by phenobarbital. Nature (New Biology) 233: 181–182 (1971).

Payne, J.P.; Hill, D.W. and King, N.W.: Observations on the distribution of alcohol in blood, breath and urine. Brit. Med. J. 1: 196–202 (1966).

Perman, E.S.: Observations on the effect of ethanol on the urinary excretion of histamine, 5-hydroxyindole acetic acid, catecholamines and 17-hydroxycorticosteroids in man. Acta Physiol. Scand. 51: 62–67 (1961).

Perman, E.S.: Increase in oxygen uptake after small ethanol doses in man. Acta Physiol. Scand. 55: 207–209 (1962a).

Perman, E.S.: Effect of ethanol on oxygen uptake and on blood glucose concentration in anesthetized rabbits. Acta Physiol. Scand. 55: 189–202 (1962b).

Perman, E.S.: Studies on the Antabuse-alcohol reaction in rabbits. Acta Physiol. Scand. 55, Suppl. 190: 5–46 (1962c).

Perman, E.S.: Intolerance to alcohol. New Eng. J. Med. 273: 114–117 (1965).

Pesch, L.A.; Segal, S. and Topper, Y.J.: Progesterone effects on galactose metabolism in prepubertal patients with congenital galactosaemia and in rats maintained on high galactose diets. J. Clin. Invest. 39: 178–184 (1960).

Peters, M.A.: Relative selectivity of some microsomal drug metabolizing enzyme inducers. Arch. Internat. Pharmacodyn. 203: 30–45 (1973).

Pieper, W.A.; Skeen, M.J.; McClure, H.M. and Bourne, P.G.: The chimpanzee as an animal model for investigating alcoholism. Science 176: 71–73 (1972).

Pietruszko, R.; Riggold, H.J.; Li, T.K.; Vallee, B.L.; Akeson, A. and Theorell, H.: Structure and function relationship in isoenzymes of horse liver alcohol dehydrogenase. Nature 221: 440–443 (1969).

Pilstrom, L. and Kiessling, K.-H.: A possible localization of α-glycerophosphate dehydrogenase to the inner boundary membrane of mitochondria in livers from rats fed with ethanol. Histochemie 32: 329–334 (1972).

Pirola, R.C. and Davis, A.E.: Effect of intravenous alcohol on motility of the duodenum and of the sphincter of Oddi. Aust. Ann. Med. 19: 24–29 (1970).

Pirola, R.C. and Lieber, C.S.: The energy cost of the metabolism of drugs, including ethanol. Pharmacology 7: 185–196 (1972).

Pirola, R.C. and Lieber, C.S.: Acute and chronic pancreatitis; Ch. 11, in Kissin and Begleiter, The Biology of Alcoholism, vol. 3: Clinical Pathology (Plenum Press, Oxford and New York 1974).

Pirola, R.C. and Lieber, C.S.: Energy wastage in rats given drugs that induce microsomal enzymes. J. Nutr. 105: 1544–1548 (1975).

Pirola, R.C. and Lieber, C.S.: Hypothesis: energy wastage in alcoholism and drug abuse; possible role of hepatic microsomal enzymes. Am. J. Clin. Nutr. 29: 90–93 (1976).

Pleuvry, B.J. and Hunter, A.R.: The effects of phenobarbitone sodium on the carbon dioxide production and oxygen consumption of the rabbit. J. Pharm. Pharmacol. 23: 19–27 (1971).

Podgainy, H. and Bressler, R.: Biochemical basis of the sulfonylurea-induced disulfiram syndrome. Diabetes 17: 679–683 (1968).

Polacsek, E.; Barnes, T.; Turner, N.; Hall, R. and Weise, C.: Interaction of alcohol and other drugs, 2nd ed. (Addiction Research Foundation, Toronto, Ontario 1972).

Portwich, F. and Aebi, H.: Erfassung der Peroxydbidung tierischer Gewebe mittels peroxydatischer Umsetzungen. Helv. Physiol. Pharmacol. Acta 18: 312–327 (1960).

Pritchard, H.M.: Economic costs of abuse and dependency on alcohol in Australia; in Kiloh and Bell, Proceedings of 29th International Congress on Alcoholism and Drug Dependence (Butterworth, Australia 1970).

Raby, K.: Relation of blood acetaldehyde levels to clinical symptoms in the disulfiram-alcohol reaction. Quart. J. Stud. Alc. 15: 21–32 (1954).

Racker, E.: Enzymatic synthesis and breakdown of desoxyribose phosphate. J. Biol. Chem. 196: 347–365 (1952).

Rajagopalan, K.V. and Handler, P.: Hepatic aldehyde oxidase. III. The substrate-binding site. J. Biol. Chem. 239: 2027–2035 (1964).

Raskin, N.H. and Sokoloff, L.: Ethanol-induced adaptation of alcohol dehydrogenase activity in rat brain. Nature 236: 138–140 (1972).

Ratcliffe, F.: The effect of chronic ethanol administration on the responses to amylobarbitone sodium in the rat. Life Sci. 8: 1051–1061 (1969).

Rawat, A.K.: Effects of ethanol infusion on the redox state and metabolic levels in rat liver in vivo. Eur. J. Biochem. 6: 585–592 (1968).

Rawat, A.K.: Effect of ethanol on glycerol metabolism in rat liver during different hormonal conditions. Biochem. Pharmacol. 19: 2791–2798 (1970).

Rawat, A.K. and Kuriyama, K.: Contribution of 'substrate shuttles' in the transport of extramitochondrial reducing equivalents by hepatic mitochondria from chronic alcohol fed mice. Arch. Biochem. Biophys. 152: 44–52 (1972).

Recknagel, R.O.: Carbon tetrachloride hepatotoxicity. Pharmacol. Rev. 19: 145–208 (1967).

Redetzki, H.M.: Alcohol-aldehyde transhydrogenation with liver alcohol dehydrogenase. Texas Reports Biol. Med. 18: 83–92 (1960).

Redmond, G. and Cohen, G.: Induction of liver acetaldehyde dehydrogenase: possible role in ethanol tolerance after exposure to barbiturates. Science 171: 387–389 (1971).

Reed, W.D. and Mezey, E.: Effects of chronic ethanol feeding on enzymes of rat brain and liver mitochondria. Life Sci. 11: 847–857 (1972).

Remmer, H.: Drugs as activators of drug enzymes; in Proceedings of the 1st International Pharmacology Meeting, vol. 6, pp.235–249 (MacMillan, New York 1962).

Remmer, H.: Induction of drug metabolizing enzymes in different animal species; in Proceedings of the European Society for the Study of Drug Toxicity, vol. 11, pp.14–18 (Excerpta Medica Foundation, Amsterdam 1969).

Remmer, H.: The induction of the enzymic 'detoxication'-system in liver cells. Rev. Can. Biol. 31: 193–222 (1972).

Remmer, H. and Merker, H.J.: Drug-induced changes in the liver endoplasmic reticulum: association with drug-metabolizing enzymes. Science 142: 1657–1658 (1963).

Remmer, H.; Schenkman, J.; Estabrook, R.W.; Sasame, H.; Gillette, J.; Narasimhulu, S.; Cooper, D.Y. and Rosenthal, O.: Drug interaction with hepatic microsomal cytochrome. Mol. Pharmacol. 2: 187–190 (1966).

Reynier, M.: Pyrazole inhibition and kinetic studies of ethanol and retinol oxidation catalyzed by rat liver alcohol dehydrogenase. Acta Chem. Scand. 23: 1119–1129 (1969).

Reynolds, E.H.: Diphenylhydantoin: Hematologic aspects of toxicity; in Woodbury, Penry and Schmidt, Antiepileptic Drugs (Raven Press, New York 1972).

Rice, C.; Orr, B. and Enquist, I.: Parenteral nutrition in the surgical patient as provided from glucose, amino acids, and alcohol. The role played by alcohol. Ann. Surgery 131: 289–306 (1950).

Riedler, G.: Einfluss des Alcohols auf die Antikoagulantientherapie. Thrombosis et Diathesis Haemorrhagica 16: 613–635 (1966).

Rinkel, M. and Myerson, A.: Alcohol absorption and intoxication; their modification by autonomic drugs. Am. J. Psych. 98: 767–769 (1942).

Ritchie, J.M.: The aliphatic alcohols; in Goodman and Gilman, The Pharmacological Basis of Therapeutics (The MacMillan Company, London and Toronto 1970).

Roach, M.K.; Khan, M.; Knapp, M. and Reese, W.N.: Ethanol metabolism in vivo and the role of hepatic microsomal ethanol oxidation. Quart. J. Stud. Alc. 33: 751–765 (1972).

Roach, M.K.; Reese, W.N. and Creaven, P.J.: Ethanol oxidation in the microsomal fraction of rat liver. Biochem. Biophys. Res. Comm. 36: 596–604 (1969).

Rodrigo, C.; Antezana, C. and Baraona, E.: Fat and nitrogen balances in rats with alcohol-induced fatty liver. J. Nutr. 101: 1307–1310 (1971).

Röe, O.: Clinical investigations of methyl alcohol poisoning with special reference to pathogenesis and treatment of amblyopia. Acta Med. Scand. 113: 558–608 (1943).

Roizin, L.: Interaction of methadone and ethanol. Presentation to the Eastern Section of American Psychiatric Association, New York (1969), quoted by Kissin (1974b).

Rubin, E. and Lieber, C.S.: Early fine structural changes in the human liver induced by alcohol. Gastroenterology 52: 1–13 (1967).

Rubin, E. and Lieber, C.S.: Alcohol-induced hepatic injury in nonalcoholic volunteers. New Eng. J. Med. 278: 869–876 (1968a).

Rubin, E. and Lieber, C.S.: Hepatic microsomal enzymes in man and rat: induction and inhibition by ethanol. Science 162: 690–691 (1968b).

Rubin, E. and Lieber, C.S.: Fatty liver, alcoholic hepatitis and cirrhosis produced by alcohol in primates. New Eng. J. Med. 290: 128–135 (1974).

Rubin, E.; Bacchin, P.; Gang, H. and Lieber, C.S.: Induction and inhibition of hepatic microsomal and mitochondrial enzymes by ethanol. Lab. Invest. 22: 569–580 (1970a).

Rubin, E.; Beattie, D.S. and Lieber, C.S.: Effects of ethanol on the biogenesis of mitochondrial membranes and associated mitochondrial functions. Lab. Invest. 23: 620–627 (1970).

Rubin, E.; Beattie, D.S.; Toth, A. and Lieber, C.S.: Structural and functional effects of ethanol on hepatic mitochondria. Fed. Proc. 31: 131–140 (1972).

Rubin, E.; Gang, H.; Misra, P.S. and Lieber, C.S.: Inhibition of drug metabolism by acute ethanol intoxication. Am. J. Med. 49: 801–806 (1970b).

Rubin, E.; Huttered, F. and Lieber, C.S.: Ethanol increases hepatic smooth endoplasmic reticulum and drug-metabolizing enzymes. Science 159: 1469–1470 (1968).

Rubin, E.; Lieber, C.S.; Alvares, A.P.; Levin, W. and Kuntzman, R.: Ethanol binding to hepatic microsomes: its increase by ethanol consumption. Biochem. Pharmacol. 20: 229–231 (1971).

de Saint-Blanquat, G.; Fritsch, P. and Derache, R.: Alcohol dehydrogenase activity of the gastric mucosa following administration of alcohol to the rat. Pathologie-Biologie (Paris) 20: 249–254 (1972).

Salaspuro, M.P. and Maenpaa, P.H.: Influence of ethanol on the metabolism of perfused normal, fatty and cirrhotic rat livers. Biochem. J. 100: 768–774 (1966).

Saltman, J.: The new alcoholics: Teenagers. Public Affairs Committee of New York City (1973).

Salvesen, H. and Kolberg, A.: Alcohol absorption in idiopathic steatorrhea. Acta. Med. Scand. 161: 135–142 (1958).

Santamaria, J.M.: The social implications of alcoholism. Med. J. Aust. 2: 523–528 (1972).

Saville, P.D. and Lieber, C.S.: Effect of alcohol on growth, bone density and muscle magnesium in the rat. J. Nutr. 87: 477–484 (1965).

Scheig, R.: Effects of ethanol on lipid metabolism in adipose tissue. Biochim. Biophys. Acta 248: 48–60 (1971).

Schenker, V.J.; Kissin, B.; Maynard, L.S. and Schenker, A.C.: The effects of ethanol on amine metabolism in alcoholism; in Marchel, Biochemical Factors in Alcoholism (Pergamon Press, Oxford and New York 1966).

Schenker, S.; Breen, K.J. and Hoyumpa, A.M.: Progress in hepatology. Hepatic encephalopathy: Current status. Gastroenterology 66: 121–151 (1974).

Schenkman, J.B.; Frey, I.; Remmer, H. and Estabrook, R.W.: Sex differences in drug metabolism by rat liver microsomes. Mol. Pharmacol. 3: 516–525 (1967).

Schiller, J.; Peck, R.E. and Goldberg, M.A.: Studies in alcoholism: effect of amino acids on the rate of disappearance of alcohol from the blood. Arch. Neurol. 1: 127–132 (1959).

Schoene, B.; Fleischman, R.A.; Remmer, H. and Oldershausen, H.F.V.: Determination of drug-metabolizing enzymes in needle biopsies of human liver. Eur. J. Clin. Pharmacol. 4: 65–73 (1972).

Scholz, R.; Hansen, W. and Thurman, R.G.: Interaction of mixed-function oxidation with biosynthetic processes. I. Inhibition of gluconeogenesis by aminopyrine in perfused rat livers. Eur. J. Biochem. 38: 64–72 (1973).

Seawright, A.A.; Steele, D.P. and Menrath, R.E.: Seasonal variation in hepatic microsomal oxidative metabolism in vitro and susceptibility to carbon tetrachloride in a flock of sheep. Aust. Vet. J. 48: 488–494 (1972).

Seegmiller, J.E.; Rosenbloom, F.M. and Kelley, W.N.: Enzyme defect associated with a sex-linked human neurological disorder and excessive purine synthesis. Science 155: 1682–1684 (1967).

Seidel, G. and Soehring, K.: Zur Frage de Anderung der Blutalkoholwerte durch Medikamente. Arzneimittel-Forschung 15: 472–474 (1965).

Sestoft, L.; Tonnesen, K.; Hansen, F.V. and Damgaard, S.E.: Fructose and D-glyceraldehyde metabolism in the isolated perfused pig liver. Eur. J. Biochem. 30: 542–552 (1972).

Shah, M.N.; Clancy, B.A. and Iber, F.L.: Comparison of blood clearance of ethanol and tolbutamide and the activity of hepatic ethanol-oxidizing and drug-metabolizing enzymes in chronic alcoholic subjects. Am. J. Clin. Nutr. 25: 135–139 (1972).

Shapiro, L.B.: Sodium amytal: effects on oxygen consumption rate in psychoses. Collect. & Contrib. Papers, Elgin State Hospital 2: 132–135 (1936).

Sherlock, S.: Diseases of the Liver and Biliary System, 4th ed. (Blackwell Scientific Publications, Oxford and Edinburgh 1968).

Shum, G.T. and Blair, A.H.: Aldehyde dehydrogenases in rat liver. Can. J. Biochem. 50: 741–748 (1972).

Siegers, C.-P.; Strubelt, O. and Back, G.: Inhibition by caffeine of ethanol absorption in rats. Eur. J. Pharmacol. 20: 181–187 (1972).

Singlevich, T. and Barboriak, J.J.: Ethanol and induction of microsomal drug-metabolizing enzymes in the rat. Toxicol. Appl. Pharmacol. 20: 284–290 (1971).

Smillie, W.G. and Pessoa, S.B.: Treatment of hookworm disease with carbon tetrachloride. Am. J. Hyg. 3: 34–45 (1923).

Smith, M.E.: Incorporation of ethanol-1-^{14}C into fatty acids in the normal and alloxan diabetic rat. Nature 190: 273–274 (1961).

Smith, M.E. and Newman, H.W.: The rate of ethanol metabolism in fed and fasting animals. J. Biol. Chem. 234: 1544–1549 (1959).

Smith, M.; Evans, R.; Newman, E. and Newman, H.: Psychotherapeutic agents and ethyl alcohol. Quart. J. Stud. Alc. 22: 241–249 (1961).

Smith, M.; Hopkinson, D.A. and Harris, H.: Developmental changes and polymorphism in human alcohol dehydrogenase. Ann. Human Genetics 34: 251–271 (1971).

Smith, J.W.; Seidl, L.G. and Cluff, L.E.: Studies on the epidemiology of adverse drug reactions. V. Clinical factors influencing susceptibility. Ann. Int. Med. 65: 629–640 (1966).

Smythe, C.M.; Heinemann, H.O. and Bradley, S.E.: Estimated hepatic blood flow in the dog. Amer. J. Physiol. 172: 737–742 (1953).

Sobel, B.; Jequier, E.; Sjoersdma, A. and Lovenberg, W.: Effect of catecholamines and adrenergic blocking agents on oxidative phosphorylation in rat heart mitochondria. Circulation Res. 19: 1050–1061 (1966).

Soehring, K. and Schuppel, R.: Wechselwirkungen zwischen Alkohol und Arzneimetten. Dtsh. Med. Wschr. 91: 1892–1898 (1966).

Söling, H.D.; Kohlaw, G.; Schnermann, J.; Holzer, H. and Creutzfeldt, W.: Zur bedeutung des Azetoins für die Pathogenese des Coma Hepaticum. Dtsch. Med. Wschr. 89: 457–463 (1964).

Sotaniemi, E.; Isoaho, R.; Huhti, E.; Huikko, M. and Koivisto, O.: Increased clearance of ethanol from the blood of asthmatic patients. Ann. Allergy 30: 254–257 (1972).

Spencer, R.P.; Brody, K.R. and Lutters, B.L.: Some effects of ethanol on the gastrointestinal tract. Am. J. Dig. Dis. 9: 599–604 (1964).

Steel, C.M.; O'Duffy, J. and Brown, S.S.: Clinical effects and treatment of imipramine and amitriptyline poisoning in children. Brit. Med. J. 2: 663–667 (1967).

Stotz, E.; Westerfeld, W.W. and Berg, R.L.: The metabolism of acetaldehyde with acetoin formation. J. Biol. Chem. 152: 41–50 (1944).

Strubelt, O.; Siegers, C.-P. and Breining, H.: Die akufe hepatotoxische Wirkung unterschiedlich konzentrierter Alkohollosungen bei oraler und intraperitonealer Applikation. Arch Toxikol. 29: 129–141 (1972).

Summerskill, W.H.J.; Wolfe, S.J. and Davidson, C.S.: Response to alcohol in chronic alcoholics with liver disease. Clinical, pathological and metabolic changes. Lancet 1: 335–340 (1957).

Sund, H. and Theorell, H.: Alcohol dehydrogenase; in Boyer, Lardy and Myrback, The Enzymes, vol. 7, 2nd ed. (Academic Press, New York and London 1963).

Sutherland, V.C.; Burbridge, T.N. and Simon, A.: Cerebral metabolism in problem drinkers under the influence of alcohol and chlorpromazine hydrochloride. J. Appl. Physiol. 15: 189–192 (1960).

Swidler, G.: Handbook of Drug Interactions (Wiley-Interscience, New York 1971).

Tephly, T.R.; Parks, R.E. and Mannering, G.J.: Methanol metabolism in the rat. J. Pharmacol. Exper. Therap. 143: 292–300 (1964).

Tephly, T.R.; Tinelli, F. and Watkins, W.D.: Alcohol metabolism: role of microsomal oxidation in vivo. Science 166: 627–628 (1969).

Teschke, R.; Hasumura, Y.; Joly, J.-G.; Ishii, H. and Lieber, C.S.: Microsomal ethanol oxidizing system (MEOS): purification and properties of a rat liver system free of catalase and alcohol dehydrogenase. Biochem. Biophys. Res. Comm. 49: 1187–1193 (1972).

Teschke, R.; Hasumura, Y. and Lieber, C.S.: Hepatic microsomal ethanol oxidizing system: solubilization, isolation and characterization. Arch. Biochem. Biophys. 163: 404–415 (1974a).

Teschke, R.; Hasumura, Y. and Lieber, C.S.: NADPH-dependent oxidation of methanol, ethanol, propranol and butanol by hepatic microsomes. Biochem. Biophys. Res. Comm. 60: 851–857 (1974b).

Theorell, H.: Alkoholdehydrogenase. Ihre Wirkungsweisen und Komplexverbindungen. Experientia (Basel) 21: 553–564 (1965).

Theorell, H.: Function and structure of liver alcohol dehydrogenase. The Harvey Lectures. Series 61, New York, pp.17–42 (1967).

Theorell, H.; Taniguchi, S.; Akeson, A. and Skursky, L.: Crystallization of a separate steroid-active liver alcohol dehydrogenase. Biochem. Biophys. Res. Comm. 24: 603–610 (1966).

Theorell, H.; Chance, B.; Yonetani, T. and Oshino, N.: The combustion of alcohol and its inhibition by 4-methyl-pyrazole in perfused rat livers. Arch. Biochem. Biophys. 151: 434–438 (1972).

Thieden, H.I.D. and Lundquist, F.: The influence of fructose and its metabolites on ethanol metabolism in vitro. Biochem. J. 102: 177–180 (1967).

Thoenen, H.; Hoefely, W.; Gey, K.F. and Huerlimann, A.: Quantitative aspects of the replacement of norepinephrine by dopamine as a sympathetic transmitter after inhibition of dopamine-β-hydroxylase by disulphiram. J. Pharmacol. Exp. Therap. 156: 246–251 (1967).

Thurman, R.G. and Scholz, R.: The role of hydrogen peroxide and catalase in hepatic microsomal ethanol oxidation. Drug. Metab. Disp. 1: 441–448 (1973).

Thurman, R.G.; Ley, H.G. and Scholz, R.: Hepatic microsomal ethanol oxidation and the role of catalase. Eur. J. Biochem. 25: 420–430 (1972).

Tipton, D.L.; Sutherland, V.C.; Burbridge, T.N. and Simon, A.: Effect of chlorpromazine on blood level of alcohol in rabbits. Amer. J. Physiol. 200: 1007–1011 (1961).

Toth, A.; Beattie, D.S.; Lieber, C.S. and Rubin, E.: Effects of ethanol on fatty acid oxidation by isolated hepatic mitochondria. Fed. Proc. 30: 573 (1971).

Trapnell, J.: The natural history and management of acute pancreatitis. Clin. Gastroenterol. 1: 147–166, H.T. Howat, ed., The Exocrine Pancreas (W.B. Saunders Co. Ltd, London 1972).

Travell, J.: The influence of the hydrogen ion concentration on the absorption of alkaloids from the stomach. J. Pharmacol. Exp. Therap. 69: 21–33 (1940).

Trémolières, J. and Carré, L.: Mise en evidence de systèmes peroxidasiques, oxydant l'alcool chez l'alcoolique. Comp. Rend. Acad. Sci. 251: 2785–2787 (1960).

Trémolières, J. and Carré, L.: Etudes sur les modalités d'oxydation de l'alcool chez l'homme normal et alcoolique. Rev. Alc. 7: 202–227 (1961).

Trémolières, J.; Lowy, R. and Griffaton, G.: Physiologie de l'oxydation et de l'utilisation de l'éthanol à doses normales et toxiques. Ann. Nutr. 21: 69–103 (1967).

Truitt, E.B. and Walsh, M.J.: The role of acetaldehyde in the actions of ethanol; in Kissin and Begleiter, The Biology of Alcoholism, vol. 1: Biochemistry (Plenum Press, New York 1971).

Truitt, E.B.; Duritz, G.; Morgan, A.M. and Prouty, R.W.: Disulfiram-like actions produced by hypoglycemic sulfonylurea compounds. Quart. J. Stud. Alc. 23: 197–207 (1962).

Tygstrup, N. and Lundquist, F.: The effect of ethanol on galactose elimination in humans. J. Lab. Clin. Med. 59: 102–109 (1962).

Uehleke, H. and Greim, H.: Stimulierung der Oxydation von Fremdstoffen in Nierenmikrosomen durch Phenobarbital. Archiv Pharmakol. Exp. Path. 261: 152–161 (1968).

Ugarte, G.; Pereda, T.; Pino, M.E. and Iturriaga, H.: Influence of alcohol intake, length of abstinence and meprobamate on the rate of ethanol metabolism in man. Quart J. Stud. Alc. 330: 698–705 (1972).

Van Eys, J.: Aldehyde-ketone isomerization activity of liver alcohol dehydrogenase. J. Biol. Chem. 236: 1531–1544 (1961).

Van Slyke, D.D. and Plamer, W.W.: Studies of acidosis; Titration of organic acids in urine. J. Biol. Chem. 41: 567–575 (1920).

Veech, R.L.; Eggleston, L.V. and Krebs, H.A.: The redox state of free nicotinamide adenine dinucleotide phosphate in the cytoplasm of rat liver. Biochem. J. 115: 609–619 (1969).

Venho, I.; Eerola, R.; Venho, E.V. and Vartiainen, O.: Sensitization to morphine by experimentally induced alcoholism in white mice. Ann. Med. Exp. Biol. Fenn 33: 249–252 (1955).

Verron, G.: Vergleischende Untershuchungen über den Sorbitolstoffweschel mit und ohne Alkoholzusatz. Z. Ges. Inn. Med. Ihre Grenz. 20: 278–283 (1965).

Vesell, E.S.: Factors altering the responsiveness of mice to hexobarbital. Pharmacology 1: 81–97 (1968).

Vesell, E.: Recent progress in pharmacogenetics. Adv. Pharmacol. Chemother. 7: 1–52 (1969).

Vesell, E.S.; Lang, C.M.; White, W.J.; Passananti, G.T. and Tripp, S.L.: Hepatic drug metabolism in rats: impairment in a dirty environment. Science 179: 896–897 (1973).

Vesell, E.S.; Page, J.G. and Passananti, G.T.: Genetic and environmental factors affecting ethanol metabolism in man. Clin. Pharmacol. Therap. 12: 192–201 (1971).

Videla, L. and Israel, Y.: Factors that modify the metabolism of ethanol in rat liver and adaptive changes produced by its chronic administration. Biochem. J. 118: 275–281 (1970).

Vitale, J.J. and Coffey, J.: Alcohol and vitamin metabolism; Ch. 10, in Kissin and Begleiter, The Biology of Alcoholism, vol. 1: Biochemistry (Plenum Press, New York 1971).

Vogel, W.H.; Snyder, R. and Schulman, M.P.: Inhibition of alcohol dehydrogenase by folic acid and several of its analogs. Proc. Soc. Exp. Biol. Med. 115: 545–549 (1964).

Wacker, W.E.C.; Haynes, H.; Druyan, R.; Fisher, W. and Coleman, J.E.: Treatment of ethylene glycol poisoning with ethyl alcohol. J. Am. Med. Ass. 194: 1231–1235 (1965).

Wada, F.; Hirata, K.; Shibata, H.; Higashi, K. and Sakamoto, Y.: Involvement of P-450 in several reactions of lipid metabolism in liver microsomes. J. Biochem. 62: 134–136 (1967).

Wagner, H.J.: The influence of various drugs and subsequent ingestion of alcohol on the metabolism. Dtsch. Z. Ger. Med. 46: 575–582 (1957).

Walker, G.W. and Curry, A.S.: 'Endogenous' alcohol in body fluids. Nature 210: 1368 (1966).

Walker, J.E.C. and Gordon, E.R.: Biochemical aspects associated with an ethanol induced fatty liver. Biochem. J. 119: 511–516 (1970).

Wallenfels, K. and Sund, H.: Über den Mechanismus der Wasserstoffubertragung mit Pyridinnucleotiden. IV. Hemmstoffe für DPN-abhängige Zinkenzyme. Biochem. Z. 329: 48–58 (1957).

Wallgren, H. and Barry, H.L.: Actions of Alcohol. Biochemical, Physiological and Psychological Aspects (Elsevier Publishing Co., Amsterdam 1970).

Walsh, M.J. and Truitt, E.B.: Release of 7-H^3-norepinephrine in plasma and urine by acetaldehyde and ethanol in cats and rabbits. Fed. Proc. 27: 601 (1968).

Walsh, M.J.; Hollander, P.B. and Truitt, E.B.: Sympathomimetic effects of acetaldehyde on the electrical and contractile characteristics of isolated left atria of guinea pigs. J. Pharmacol. Exp. Therap. 167: 173–186 (1969).

Waltman, R.; Bonura, F.; Nigrin, G. and Pipat, C.: Ethanol in prevention of hyperbilirubinaemia in the newborn. Lancet 2: 1265–1267 (1969).

Von Wartburg, J.-P.: The metabolism of alcohol in normals and alcoholics: Enzymes; in Kissin and Begleiter, The Biology of Alcoholism, vol. 1: Biochemistry (Plenum Press, New York and London 1971).

Von Wartburg, J.-P. and Eppenberger, H.M.: Vergleichende Untersuchungen über den oxydativen Abbau von l-C^{14}-Äthanol und l-C^{14}-Azetat in Leber und Niere. Helv. Physiol. Pharmacol. Acta 19: 303–322 (1961).

Von Wartburg, J.-P. and Papenberg, J.: Alcohol dehydrogenase in ethanol metabolism. Psychosom. Med. 28: 405–413 (1966).

Von Wartburg, J.-P. and Rothlisberger, M.: Enzymatische Veranderungen in der Leber nach landauernder Belastung mit Aethanol und Methanol bei der Ratte. Helv. Physiol. Pharmacol. Acta 19: 30–41 (1961).

Von Wartburg, J.-P.; and Schurch, P.M.: A typical human liver alcohol dehydrogenase. Ann. N.Y. Acad. Sci. 151: 936–946 (1968).

Von Wartburg, J.-P.; Papenberg, J. and Aebi, H.: An atypical human alcohol dehydrogenase. Can. J. Biochem. 43: 889–898 (1965).

Von Wartburg, J.-P.; Bethune, J.L. and Vallee, B.L.: Purification and enzymatic properties of human liver alcohol dehydrogenase. American Chemical Society, 143rd Meeting, Abstracts, 100c (1963).

Von Wartburg, J.-P. Bethune, J.L. and Vallee, B.L.: Human liver alcohol dehydrogenase. Kinetic and physicochemical properties. Biochemistry 3: 1775–1782 (1964).

Watanabe, T.; Sato, M. and Ide, T.: Studies on alcohol poisoning using ethanol-l-^{14}C in mice. Japan. Stud. Alc. 1: 165–179 (1966), quoted by Wallgren and Barry (1970).

Wattenberg, L.W. and Leong, J.L.: Histochemical demonstration of reduced pyridine nucleotide dependent polycyclic hydrocarbon-metabolizing systems. J. Histochem. Cytochem. 10: 412–420 (1962).

Wattenberg, L.W. and Leong, J.L.: Effects of phenothiazines on protective systems against polycyclic hydrocarbons. Cancer Research 25: 365–370 (1965).

Wattenberg, L.W.; Leong, J.L. and Strand, P.J.: Benzpyrene hydroxylase activity in the gastrointestinal tract. Cancer Research 22: 1120–1125 (1962).

Watts, D.T. and Gourley, D.R.H.: A simple apparatus for determining basal metabolism of small animals in a student laboratory. Proceedings of the Society for Biological and Experimental Medicine 84: 585–586 (1953).

Weiner, H.: The role of zinc in liver alcohol dehydrogenase; in Sardesai, Biochemical and Clinical Aspects of Alcohol Metabolism (Charles C. Thomas, Springfield, Ill. 1969).

Weiss, R. and Reiss, M.: Über die Wirkung des Alkohols auf den respiratorischen Stoff-wechsel. Z. Ges. Exp. Med. 38: 420–427 (1923).

Welch, R.M.; Harrison, Y.; Gommi, B.W.; Poppers, P.J.; Finster, M. and Conney, A.H.: Stimulatory effect of cigarette smoking on the hydroxylation of 3,4-benzpyrene and the N-demethylation of 3-methyl-4-monomethylaminoazobenzene by enzymes in human placenta. Clin. Pharm. Ther. 10: 100–109 (1969).

Werk, E.E.; MacGee, J. and Sholiton, L.J.: Effect of diphenylhydantoin on cortisol metabolism in man. J. Clin. Invest. 43: 1824–1835 (1964).

Werk, E.E.; Sholiton, L.J. and Olinger, C.P.: Amelioration of non-tumorous Cushing's syndrome by diphenylhydantoin. 2nd International Congress on Hormonal Steroids, Milan; in Abstracts, International Congress Series No. 111, p.301 (Excerpta Medica Foundation, New York 1966).

Whitfield, J.B.; Moss, D.W.; Neale, G.; Orme, M. and Breckenridge, A.: Changes in plasma Δ-glutamyl transpeptidase activity associated with alterations in drug metabolism in man. Brit. Med. J. 1: 316–318 (1973).

Whittlesey, P.: The effect of pentobarbital on the metabolism of ethyl alcohol in dogs. Bulletin of the Johns Hopkins Hospital 95: 81–89 (1954).

Widmark, E.M.P.: Über die Konzentration des genossenen Alkohols in Blut und Harn unter verschiedenen Umständen. Skand. Arch. Physiol. 33: 85–107 (1915).

Wilhelmj, C.M.; Bollman, J.L. and Mann, F.C.: Studies on the physiology of the liver. The effect of removal of the liver on the specific dynamic action of amino acids admin-istered intravenously. Am. J. Physiol. 87: 497–509 (1928).

Wilkinson, P.; Kornaczewski, A.; Rankin, J.G. and Santamaria, J.N.: Physical disease in alcoholism. Initial survey of 1000 patients. Med. J. Aust. 1: 1217–1227 (1971).

Williams, E.E.: Effects of alcohol on workers with carbon disulfide. J. Am. Med. Ass. 109: 1472–1473 (1937).

Williams, R.T.: Thalidomide. A study of biochemical teratology. Arch. Envir. Health 16: 493–502 (1968).

Williams, R.T.: Hepatic metabolism of drugs. Gut 13: 579–585 (1972).

Wilson, G.M.: Ill-health due to drugs. Brit. Med. J. 1: 1065–1069 (1966).

Wilson, R.H.L.; Newman, E.J. and Newman, H.W.: Diurnal variation in rate of alcohol metabolism. J. Appl. Physiol. 8: 556–558 (1956).

Winkler, K.; Tygstrup, N. and Lundquist, F.: The influence of fructose on the hepatic circulation and metabolism in man. Acta Physiol. Scand. 59, Suppl. 213: p.167 (1963).

Winne, D. and Remischovsky, J.: Der Einfluss der Durchblutung auf die Resorption von Harnstoff, Methanol und Äthanol aus dem Jejunum der Ratte. Naunyn-Schmiedeberg Archiv Pharmakol. 268: 392–416 (1971).

Wolff, P.H.: Ethnic differences in alcohol sensitivity. Science 175: 449–450 (1972).

Woodward, E.R.; Robertson, C.; Ruttenberg, H.D. and Schapiro, H.: Alcohol as a gastric secretory stimulant. Gastroenterology 32: 727–737 (1957).

Yesair, D.W.; Bullock, F.J. and Coffey, J.: The pharmacodynamics of drug interaction. Drug. Metab. Rev. 1: 35–70 (1972).

Ylikahri, R.H.; Hassinen, I.E. and Kähönen, M.T.: Metabolic interactions of fructose and ethanol in perfused liver of normal and thyroxine-treated rats. Metabolism 20: 555–567 (1971).

Ziegler, D.M.; Mitchell, C.H. and Jollow, D.: The properties of a purified hepatic micro-somal mixed function amine oxidase; in Gillette, Conney, Cosmides, Estabrook, Fouts and Mannering, Microsomes and Drug Oxidations, pp.173–188 (Academic Press, New York 1969).

Zilly, W.; Brachtel, D. and Richter, E.: Hexobarbitalplasmaspiegel bei Patienten mit akuter Hepatitis während kontinuierlicher Hexobarbital-Infusion. Klin. Wschr. 51: 346–347 (1973).

Zirkle, G.A.; King, P.D.; McAtee, O.B. and Van Dyke, R.: Effects of chlorpromazine and alcohol on coordination and judgement. J. Am. Med. Ass. 171: 1496–1499 (1959).

Zuppinger, K.; Papenberg, J.; Schürch, P.; Von Wartburg, J.-P.; Colombo, J.P. and Rossi, E.: Vermehrte Alkoholoxydation bei der Glykogenose Typ I. Schweiz. Med. Wschr. 97: 1110–1117 (1967).

Subject Index